Praise for *The Drive At 35* and Andy Lipman

An MVP Expresses Gratitude

Andy Lipman gives all who read *The Drive at 35* a new perspective for thinking about our approach to life, and how to tackle life's most difficult challenges. Early on in my career with the Atlanta Braves, I was honored to be a spokesman for the local chapter of the 65 Roses Club, a charity dedicated to raising money for the Cystic Fibrosis Foundation and increasing awareness about the multifaceted challenges of this disease. Getting to know people with CF opened my eyes. These individuals faced their situations with courage and strength. I've always remembered their examples to me.

Andy Lipman faces life with that same courage and strength, and it allows him to meet the challenges of CF head on. He is fearless and optimistic. This isn't to say he doesn't have periods of doubt and concern, but we can all learn from his example as he addresses these times. He is open and honest in *The Drive at 35*, and its pages will inspire you to live your life to the fullest. This is a book for everyone. Andy stands as a role model and guide for all of us as we go down life's paths. Andy says, "Here is how you do it. I did it and so can you."

I would like to say, "Thank you, Andy!" You give all of us an understanding of what it means to truly live our dreams and to love our lives, regardless of the challenges we face. Thank you. Thanks for helping all of us live and love more deeply and more meaningfully.

All my best,
Dale Murphy
Atlanta Braves #3. 1976-1990
NL MVP '82, '83

A Blurb from Boomer

People with cystic fibrosis are living longer and enjoying a better quality of life. In fact, over 40 percent of people with cystic fibrosis are living into adulthood. Andy Lipman, who is living, breathing and succeeding at thirty-five with CF, raises awareness of this life threatening disease, and serves as a mentor giving hope to individuals living with CF and their families.

Truly inspirational, Andy's story shows everyone that despite obstacles, life is for living and truly worth it.

Sincerely,
Boomer Esiason
Former NFL All-Pro Quarterback and CBS Sports Commentator

* * * * * * *

An Open Letter of Appreciation

On behalf of the Cystic Fibrosis Foundation, I am pleased to convey my appreciation for your tireless efforts in support of our mission to control and cure cystic fibrosis. From the A Wish for Wendy softball tournament to the CF CureFinders fundraiser and the many other events in which you volunteer substantial time and effort you have done so much to help the Foundation serve the CF community.

Because of dedicated volunteers like you, we have made significant strides toward fulfilling our mission and improving the quality of life for those with the disease.

You should be extremely proud of all you have accomplished, in honor of your sister and in support of everyone in the CF community. Please know that your significant contributions over the years have helped bring hope and optimism to all those affected by this disease.

I am honored to partner with you as we work together toward a cure for CF. Thanks for all you do.

Sincerely,
Robert Beall, President & CEO
Cystic Fibrosis Foundation

THE DRIVE AT 35

The Long Road to Beating Cystic Fibrosis

Andy Lipman

Foreword by Céline Dion

Preface by Garth Brooks

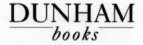

The Drive At 35 © 2011 by Andy Lipman

Published in Nashville, Tennessee by Dunham Books.

For information on licensing and special sales, please contact:

Dunham Books
63 Music Square East
Nashville, Tennessee 37203
www.dunhamgroupinc.com

ISBN 978-0-9837-4569-3
Ebook ISBN 978-0-9839-9061-1

Printed in the United States of America

Dedication

This book is dedicated to my wife, my parents, my sister, and the rest of my family for sticking by me. When the going got tough, you didn't give up on me. I'd also like to dedicate this book to Dr. Thomas Boat, my physician for nearly two decades. You are not only a wonderful doctor, but a great friend as well. And to Avery and Ethan, thanks for making my biggest dream come true.

Table of Contents

Praise for *The Drive At 35* and Andy Lipman i

Foreword by Céline Dion 1

Preface by Garth Brooks 3

A Message from Andy 5

Introduction by Frank Deford 7

Chapter One: The Poster 9

Chapter Two: Not Your "Average" Kid 11

Chapter Three: The Enemy Exposed 19

Chapter Four: My Father, My Hero 23

Chapter Five: Finding Fire Through Sports 29

Chapter Six: Man's Best Friend 33

Chapter Seven: The Best and Worst of Being Twelve 37

Chapter Eight: Running on Empty 41

Chapter Nine: A Rescue Boat 45

Chapter Ten: My Partner in Crime 49

Chapter Eleven: A Rush Decision 55

Chapter Twelve: Extreme Makeover—Andy Edition 59

Chapter Thirteen: Scared to be Different 65

Chapter Fourteen: CF Stands for "Crutch Found" 69

Chapter Fifteen: Doctor Doom 73

Chapter Sixteen: A Nightmarish Return 77

Chapter Seventeen: The Final Straw 81

Chapter Eighteen: Knocked Down…But not Out 85

Chapter Nineteen: Getting a Huge Weight Off My Chest 89

Chapter Twenty: Picking My Moment 95

Chapter Twenty-One: CF Attacks…But not in the Lungs 101

Chapter Twenty-Two: A Reason to Run 107

Chapter Twenty-Three: Meeting Wendy 113

Chapter Twenty-Four: What Am I About? 119

Chapter Twenty-Five: A Wish Comes True 125

Chapter Twenty-Six: Who Was That Girl? 129

Chapter Twenty-Seven: The One 131

Chapter Twenty-Eight: The Ultimate Honor 137

Chapter Twenty-Nine: A New Group of Friends 141

Chapter Thirty: Slim to None 145

Chapter Thirty-One: The "Other" Club 1150 149

Chapter Thirty-Two: A Little Magic in Our Lives 157

Chapter Thirty-Three: Third Time's a Charm? 161

Chapter Thirty-Four: A Difficult Pregnancy for Dad 165

Chapter Thirty-Five: Parenting CF Style 171

Chapter Thirty-Six: A Normal Day at the Doctor's Office 175

Chapter Thirty-Seven: Getting the Picture 179

Chapter Thirty-Eight: Trying for Baby Number Two 183

Chapter Thirty-Nine: First Blood 189

Chapter Forty: Rearing Its Ugly Head 195

Chapter Forty-One: Struggling to Find Strength 199

Chapter Forty-Two: The Enigma 207

Chapter Forty-Three: Not Afraid to Tri! 215

Chapter Forty-Four: My Other CF Symptom 219

Chapter Forty-Five: Wishing I Was More Rusty 231

Epilogue 235

About the Author 239

Foreword

I was honored to be asked to provide the Foreword for this moving memoir. *The Drive at 35* is such an inspiring account of Andy Lipman's life with cystic fibrosis. It is also the candid story of a young man finding his way in the world, despite big challenges.

Known today as the most common, fatal genetic disease affecting young persons throughout North America, cystic fibrosis (CF) attacks both breathing and digestion. Research funded by charitable donations has made it possible for children and adults with CF to live longer and healthier lives. Yet, so far, a cure has eluded us.

Cystic fibrosis has also touched my life in a very personal way. My beloved niece, Karine, lost her battle with CF at the age of sixteen. Like Andy, I remain committed to doing all I can to help defeat this devastating disease, which is still stealing the future from so many young people.

The Drive at 35 is Andy's journey, but one he has not had to make alone. Through his reflections, we are privileged to revisit the highs and lows of his life, and to celebrate two of life's miracles—the birth of his daughter, Avery, and son Ethan. As a parent, I know the great joy that children can bring. I wish Andy, his wife Andrea, Avery and Ethan many, many happy years together.

On behalf of the Canadian Cystic Fibrosis Foundation, and the families who battle CF bravely every day, I would like to thank Andy Lipman for supporting the cause we share by raising awareness of this fatal disease, and for supporting the Canadian Cystic Fibrosis Foundation with a donation from the proceeds of this book.

I remain confident that together, we will beat cystic fibrosis, once and for all. And as Andy says, I know that CF will one day stand for "cure found."

— **Céline Dion**
Celebrity Patron for the Canadian Cystic Fibrosis Foundation

Preface

Albert Einstein once said, "The only source of knowledge is experience..." and when it comes to the devastating illness of cystic fibrosis, Andy Lipman knows what he is talking about. From the tragic passing of his sister, Wendy, to his own everyday head-to-head battle with CF, Andy has experienced the disease on all levels and he has persevered.

Using his experience and following his heart, Andy started the "Wish for Wendy Foundation" to not only help find a cure but to remind all of us that his sister is still fighting this disease. Andy has personally taken on the success of the foundation, which has already passed the seven-figure mark with no signs of slowing down. This book is no different, as royalties from the sales of *The Drive at 35* will go to the Cystic Fibrosis Foundation in all of its efforts to cure CF. It takes a special human being to take on such a challenge, but I know his family and trust me, "special" is in their blood.

— **Garth Brooks, International Recording Artist**

A Message from Andy

My name is Andy Lipman and I have cystic fibrosis . . . but it will never have me. Or, should I say, it will never have me again. Cystic fibrosis has controlled my life on and off for many years, but I don't intend for this disease to win the war.

Most people know very little about cystic fibrosis. When I give talks about CF, the response I hear most often is, "I've heard of it, but I just don't know much about it."

Cystic fibrosis is a genetic disease that causes a sticky buildup of mucus in the lungs, as well as pancreatic deficiency. It is a recessive disease, occurring only when a child inherits two mutated copies of the CF gene, one from each parent. When mucus builds in the lungs, breathing is extremely difficult and the risk of lung infections is much greater than for the average person. Pancreatic issues make it difficult to digest foods, requiring CF patients, more often than not, to take enzymes with their meals.

Cystic fibrosis affects more than just the digestive and respiratory systems. It also affects the reproductive system. Only two percent of men with CF can have children, because most males with CF are born without a fully formed *vas deferens*, the bridge that transfers semen to the penis. I will go into detail about the other options I had to consider in order to have children, including in vitro fertilization.

Cystic fibrosis affects seventy thousand people worldwide. In the United States, thirty thousand people live with cystic fibrosis and each year several hundred die as a result. When I was born in the early seventies, life expectancy for those with CF was in the teens. Research and the development of new drugs, made possible through the fundraising efforts of the Cystic Fibrosis Foundation and other organizations, has ensured that the median expected age increases every year. Today, it is in the late thirties. Still, there is currently no cure for cystic fibrosis.

Despite the advances, brave children and adults battle this disease every day, some fully aware of their prognosis, others too young to understand. Some are in stable condition; others more critical. All of us have one thing in common, though. We all hope for more effective treatments and eventually a cure for this horrible disease.

For the most part, I have been fortunate. I have staved off infections, work a full-time job and have a relatively normal life. Some of that is due to luck, but a lot can be credited to hard work. If this book demonstrates anything, it is that we can make choices that create amazing differences in our lives. Plus, dreams, however difficult to understand, can be a great source of motivation. Mine have helped me learn to live my life with great passion and to love every minute of it.

When I began writing *The Drive at 35*, I knew I had a story that could help others, so I made sure the book did not pull any punches. *The Drive at 35* is my declaration that every book and doctor that told me I could not live past the age of twenty-five was wrong. I also wanted to tell more than the story of a competitive person with a life-threatening disease. I wanted to tell the story of a person with hopes and dreams—just like everyone else—but who must also deal with extraordinary circumstances. CF isn't just a disease that affects the lungs; it also affects a person's attitude and emotions. I'm not any different. While I have done many positive things in my life, I've also made plenty of mistakes and gone through tough times like any other human being. In particular, I have dealt with depression most of my life and it has negatively affected my loved ones. Much of this can be attributed to the trauma I encountered as a young boy. This book does not shy away from those unpleasant times.

My purpose is to raise awareness about cystic fibrosis and help fund cystic fibrosis research. This book shares a story that proves determination can defeat even the most challenging foes. A percentage of the proceeds will help fund cystic fibrosis research, so the fact you are reading it means you are helping, too.

Thank you so very much for your support.

— **Andy Lipman**
Cystic fibrosis survivor of thirty-five years and counting

Introduction

Andy Lipman's sister, Wendy, lived just two weeks before she succumbed to cystic fibrosis. When Andy was born with the disease a few years later, in 1973, his life expectancy was about ten years. I know this only too well, because my own daughter, Alex, was born with CF in 1971 and lived only eight years.

Andy beat the odds. In a way, he has swum out with the ebb tide, for as the life expectancy of people with cystic fibrosis has increased year by year, so has his own life. Today, he is living a full life as a husband and father at the age of thirty-five—and that age is about the life span that can be predicted for the average person with this terrible disease.

That, of course, is a wonderful advance, but although Andy's life is so much longer than the one that was anticipated for him, living with CF is never easy, no matter how many the years. It's like what the great champion, Joe Louis, said about a quicker opponent: "He can run, but he can't hide." No matter how well Andy manages to live, no matter how hard he fights, no matter how much he outdistances the sentence he was given, he never gets completely away from cystic fibrosis. It's always a struggle.

This, then, is his story of how, at an age he was never supposed to reach, Andy Lipman battles on courageously with enthusiasm and nobility and hope and a love of life that can inspire us all.

— **Frank Deford**
Sports Illustrated, NPR, & HBO's *Real Sports* Commentator

Chapter 1
The Poster

The year was 1981. The first test tube baby was born in the United States, Sandra Day O'Connor became the first female U.S. Supreme Court Justice, and a new cable channel called MTV debuted. While the world was introduced to these firsts, breakthroughs in the study of cystic fibrosis were few and far between. Role models beating CF were non-existent. The median life expectancy for those battling the disease was in the teens, and a cure remained elusive.

I was eight years old in 1981. I knew very little about cystic fibrosis back then and nothing about my life expectancy. I was a skinny kid who coughed a lot, but I never thought too much about it. I took medication and endured therapies, but didn't understand that if I didn't do these things I would die. My parents were very careful to keep information about this genetic disease from me. They believed such knowledge would cause overwhelming fear.

My mother regularly took me to a specialist who treated cystic fibrosis patients. I was constantly getting bad news from him and recall one specific day when Dr. Caplan was especially worried about my cough. I'd had a lot of doctor's appointments, but rarely one where the doctor and my mother looked so concerned. I'd never been more afraid in my entire life.

The nurse took me to have a sputum culture. I spit in a jar and the nurse sent the mucous to a lab where it was tested to see what kind of bacteria was in my system. From this, the doctor determined what kind of antibiotics should help. Mom heard me hacking from four rooms over and came running. She was perplexed as to why none of the meds I was taking were helping. What was wrong with me, I wondered. Why was I always so sick? Would I always feel this way?

As we returned, something caught my attention. I stopped in front of a large advertisement for a weight-gain drink featuring an extraordinary athlete. He was shirtless and muscular, easily the most physically fit person I'd ever seen. He was flexing his muscles and smiling with unmistakable confidence. I kept staring at him and my mom noticed.

"He has cystic fibrosis," she said. "Look how strong he is. You can look just like him."

At that moment this poster became something more than just a random picture. This was no ordinary man. He did the same treatments I did. He took the same meds I took. He probably saw the same doctors. I wondered if he played football or was a pro wrestler. Either way, he persevered using the same routines I did. I made up my mind then and there that I would grow to have his confidence and someday be able to flex my muscles just like he did. I wasn't going to feel sick forever. I was going to meet this guy someday and thank him for inspiring me. In an instant, this nameless man became my role model.

Seeing that hulking figure on the wall removed many of my fears about cystic fibrosis. In the following years, I looked for the poster every time I visited my doctor. Seeing the poster was the single highlight of every appointment. One day, it was gone. I never found out who he was, but the man with the muscular arms and enormous chest had done his job. He had changed my attitude and that new attitude saved my life.

Chapter 2
Not Your "Average" Kid

From the moment I was born at a whopping ten pounds, ten ounces on September 4, 1973, I was thrust into the underdog role. Because my sister Wendy had cystic fibrosis, doctors knew I had a one in four chance of having it, too. The only way to get cystic fibrosis is if both parents have the CF gene and, unfortunately, mine did. This was before prenatal screening, so there was no way of knowing that Wendy or I had the disease.

I was a strong baby. My Aunt Susie claimed I kicked myself across the entire warming tray right after I was born. She and my father were the first ones to see me, as my mother was sedated during the procedure. My father noticed almost immediately that I had a distended belly, a symptom of cystic fibrosis. Once the doctors concurred, my parents knew that I, like my sister, would have to battle a life-threatening disease all my life.

My aunt remembers the moment when my father got down on his knees, reached for my mother's hand and whispered to her that, like my sister, I had cystic fibrosis.

"Watching his face close to hers, both of them crying, was a moment that really broke my heart," she said.

Soon after I was born, I was taken by ambulance to Egleston Children's Hospital in Atlanta, where the doctors cleared my blocked intestine. At the time Egleston had only one CF specialist, Dr. Daniel Caplan, who became my doctor. From him, and their previous experience with my sister, my parents learned that other problems newborns with cystic fibrosis typically have include failure to grow, bulky and greasy stools, and frequent respiratory infections.

On the eighth day of life, it is Jewish tradition that young males be circumcised by a mohel, who is specifically trained to perform the circumcision. My operation, however, was performed by a doctor at the hospital. I still had a celebration bris eight days after my birth, where my parents showed me off, but because the risk of exposure to germs could be fatal to me, my appearance was fairly brief. Many guests were nervous, but along with the rabbi, they prayed I would have a long and healthy life.

Three years earlier, my sister had passed away just sixteen days after her birth. While I knew I had a sister, my parents never told me how Wendy died. For many years I was naïve and thought she had succumbed to Sudden Infant Death Syndrome (SIDS) or some other childhood disease. It wasn't until I was twenty-five years old that I found out how Wendy died.

Neither did I know my doctors believed I'd be fortunate if I reached my teens. My parents tried to remain optimistic. They wrote letters to doctors in New Zealand, who were working on a new treatment for CF. Nothing ever came of it, though. They also corresponded with research doctors at the University of Calgary in Alberta, Canada, but these doctors were very secretive about their work and the trials never reached completion. My parents were quite willing to sell their home and move to New Zealand or Canada if they could find a place that would give me a better quality of life. Unfortunately, there were no major breakthroughs.

Growing up in Doraville, a small suburb a few miles north of Atlanta, in many ways I was like most kids. I loved to watch television, I hated eating spinach and I didn't like going to school. I wanted more than anything to be a normal kid, but the fact was, I never would be. Cystic fibrosis robbed me of normalcy the moment I was born.

My parents were always concerned about my health. If one of them got sick, my mom or dad immediately went to their room and remained quarantined till the cold was gone. There were occasions when my dad wore a mask because he worried he might give me something. At school, teachers were told to watch out for me and make sure I took my medications before I ate lunch. All this was because the immune system of someone with cystic fibrosis is impaired. For most people, it takes a week to get rid of a cold. For me, it could take a month. That's if the cold didn't turn into something worse. Then I could die.

At home, my parents pleaded with me to eat, as if eating would cure me of cystic fibrosis. But I hated to eat. Eating made me feel like I was taking a standardized test every night. My mom counted down the number of pieces of chicken I had left as if she were Dick Clark and we were waiting for the ball to drop on New Year's Eve.

My family didn't talk about cystic fibrosis when I was little. At least not in front of me. I knew it wasn't something everyone had, and I knew it wasn't something anyone wanted. Other than having my parents administer therapy—every day they had to pound my chest to release the thick mucus from my lungs—and taking two to three pills prior to each meal, I didn't think too much about it.

My parents also did my postural drainage treatments every day. These treatments loosened the phlegm in my lungs and allowed me to cough it up.

First they slipped the nebulizer mask on my face and turned on the "mist machine," as we called it, for about thirty minutes. I was supposed to sit up throughout the treatment, but I frequently fell asleep. My mom then had to come in, wake me, and make me sit up. After the mist machine, we moved to the other half-hour of therapy, which consisted of thumping on my chest to loosen the mucus. Sometimes this hurt a bit, but mostly it was just uncomfortable.

I hated my therapy because it took so much time. I remember that on family trips my cousin Barrett would race to the beach and be building sand castles or catching hermit crabs and sand dollars, while I'd have to endure an hour of therapy before getting a glimpse of sunlight. I always felt left behind. I never asked why I did the treatments or took the pills. Of course, as a child, I didn't understand much and I didn't know what to ask. Fortunately, my parents were on top of things when it came to cystic fibrosis.

When I was in grade school, my mother made what I consider to be one of the most important decisions about my life. We were at the hospital for my monthly checkup with Dr. Caplan, who looked perpetually concerned about my health. My mom called him a "pessimistic" doctor. Then again, there weren't too many doctors who were optimistic about the outlook for a kid with cystic fibrosis. That day, Dr. Caplan suggested my mom send me to cystic fibrosis camp.

This camp, I learned, was where kids with cystic fibrosis could get together and talk about CF. Unfortunately, going there also included the risk of catching a serious bacterial illness, such as pseudomonas. I'd learn much later in life that this was a potentially deadly type of bacteria that can destroy the lungs, cause respiratory failure, and is very difficult to treat. All of the potential campers were tested before they enrolled, but that was no guarantee against infection. If one camper was affected, pseudomonas could easily spread to everyone—with possibly fatal consequences.

Dr. Caplan knew this, but he told my mom that the benefits outweighed the risks. He recommended I attend the camp to meet other kids who knew how it felt to have therapy every day and learn how they handled the challenges of CF.

It sounded good to me. I just wanted to go and play with the other campers. I figured my mom would say yes.

Mom considered Dr. Caplan's recommendation carefully. She looked at me, but I don't think she was asking me to decide; she realized this wasn't about the brand of peanut butter she was going to buy. This was her son's life. Then she stunned both of us and said, "I'd prefer he didn't go. I don't want Andy to become friends with kids he'll see pass away, and I don't want him to think he's different just because he has CF. I want him to have a normal life. He deserves that opportunity."

So many times, Dr. Caplan had told my mother and me about the things I couldn't do, but on this day she was telling him that I could accomplish a lot. She wasn't going to let me be defined by CF. She wanted me to be a kid like every other kid. And while I didn't understand the importance of her decision then, I later realized that my mother, a constant worrier, had confidence in me.

Despite my huge birth weight, in grade school I became known for being small, weak and ill. To top it off, my parents didn't trust me to take my medications. It wasn't because I was a bad kid, but rather the fact that I was a kid. So every day during lunch, I went to the principal's office to get my medication. My friends obviously wondered why I went there so often and I told them that my mom left my lunch there. Without those pills, I couldn't eat lunch. So, technically, I wasn't lying.

I never revealed to anyone that I had cystic fibrosis. I knew from my pessimistic doctor's appointments that CF was nothing to brag about. If any of my peers knew that I had the disease, they most likely found out from a teacher or parent. I became adept at keeping many secrets about myself. Unfortunately, this unhealthy skill became as much a part of me as my cystic fibrosis.

Even if my classmates didn't know I had cystic fibrosis, they quickly figured out that I was such a poor athlete that no one wanted me on their team. I always finished last when we ran laps in gym class. Sometimes it took me so long that the gym teacher told me not to finish, because everyone else was ready to move on to another activity. It was absolutely humiliating. My parents, however, didn't seem too concerned about this. When I was sick, my mom would write a note to the gym teacher asking that I be excused because of cystic fibrosis. At the time, the notes were a relief. I didn't have to embarrass myself. Looking back, I wish she had never written them.

Over the years, my classmates learned that I had CF. I doubt any of them knew much about it, but as a kid, any difference is perceived as bad. I became a target. Some kids taunted me by saying I'd be dead before I ever got to high school. One girl used to grab my frail arm and say, "You're so skinny!" I'd come home many days so devastated that I cried and cried. My mom told me that everything was fine, but I didn't know who or what to believe. Mom had always been there for me, but was adamant about me taking my pills. She asked me every day after school if I had taken them. It made me realize that if I didn't, something really bad would happen, so I began to believe my classmates. More and more, I realized that I wasn't "your average kid."

I missed a lot of school when I was young. It's normal for a kid to get a sniffle, but it's far more serious for someone with cystic fibrosis. I hated being sick. Being home was worse than being picked on in school. I used to sit inside with my dog, Howard, and watch enviously as the other kids played ball outside, sometimes in my own yard. Cystic fibrosis was not just physically debilitating. It was also emotionally draining, because I felt like I could never do the normal things that other kids were able to do.

We had a great place with easily the biggest yard in the neighborhood. Both our front and backyards were flat so they were great for sports. Kids also liked skipping rocks in the creek in the back, and we had woods where some of the kids rode dirt bikes.

Howard and I often watched the neighborhood kids play, but no one ever asked me to join in. Since I'd never played sports, I couldn't blame them, but for a kid, even a sick one, it was tough always looking out the window. When my mom did let me go outside, it was with a stern warning to be careful and not overexert myself. Mom wanted me to have a life, but she had a lot of fear, too.

I spent most of my afternoons parked in front of the TV watching cartoons and sitcoms. I probably watched six hours of TV a day. I couldn't do anything else, and shows like *Diff'rent Strokes*, *The Facts of Life*, *Sanford and Son* and *The Carol Burnett Show*, with their laugh tracks and easily resolved problems, were my way of escaping reality. Unlike my dad, TV never yelled at me or expected anything from me.

Every night when my father came home, he'd ask what I'd done that day. He was never pleased to learn that I'd spent another afternoon glued to the screen.

"You need to go outside," he said. "You need to play with your friends."

As if I had any friends. No one wanted to play with me. I didn't want to tell that to my dad, though, because I thought he'd be even more disappointed in me than he already was. I often had the sense that my dad expected more from me than I knew how to give. I thought of the dads I'd seen on TV happily playing catch with their sons, dispensing wise advice and fixing everything that was wrong. I wasn't anything like those freckle-faced kids. I feared my dad regretted having such a sickly skinny kid and didn't love me. Perhaps I was disappointed, too . . . disappointed that my dad, who seemed to be able to handle any situation and fix any problem, couldn't fix me. I was his child, wasn't I? Wasn't there anything he could do? Didn't he see how unhappy I was?

Looking back, I see that my mom and dad were opposites. My mother feared for my life, but tried to remain supportive. Dad wanted me to enjoy whatever time I had, but had a poor way of motivating me. They agreed on one thing. Cystic fibrosis was not a topic that was to be discussed openly when I was in the room.

My father's poor motivational skills and my mother's fear of talking about anything related to CF were not the primary reasons my youth was difficult. I wish they were the only reasons, but unfortunately there were other components. There were things that happened to me during my early grammar school years that until now I was ashamed to mention.

When I was eight years old, a male babysitter beat me. It was awkward because I was a friend of his siblings and could never tell them what their teenage brother did to me. His reasoning for hitting me was that I would not go to bed. The most frightening part was that he always did it while we were watching *The Incredible Hulk*. It was as if he became the Hulk, and to this day I get chills when I see anything regarding the green monster.

I remember one night my parents were going to see the movie *An American Werewolf in London* and I knew he was going to babysit again. As she sat in front of the mirror to do her hair, I begged my mom not to go. But, I didn't tell her about the beatings I was going to receive because he told me he would hurt me worse if I told.

The following morning, after another abusive night, probably the worst one to date, my mother was doing my therapy when I cried out in pain. She thought her ring might have hurt me, so she took it off. Then she tried again and another scream followed. She lowered my shorts and saw the red handprints. My mom was angry and asked me what happened. I didn't want to tell because I didn't want the beatings to get worse.

She then asked, "Did the babysitter do this?" I paused in horror and nodded, knowing that my well-being was now in jeopardy. "I'm going to talk to your dad right now," she said. I never knew what happened after that. The whole thing went away. We never discussed it. The only change was that he never babysat me again. I still saw him from time to time, as he was one of my neighbors, but each time I saw him I raced to our courtyard and hid. I could not get his evil sneer out of my head. I think the secrecy of the issue affected how I coped with things as I got older. Keep quiet or risk adversity.

The babysitter's abuse was not the worst thing to happen to me. Around the time the beatings occurred, I spent several evenings at a family friend's home. The parents had three daughters. One of the daughters, whom my mom said was mentally slower than the others, used to take me upstairs. I remember her face had the distinctive flattened features of what I now believe to be a symptom of a genetic syndrome or other medical condition, and she had short blonde hair.

Once we got upstairs, she asked me to disrobe and sit with her in the nude. She took off most of her clothes, leaving only her bra and panties. I was conflicted. I was excited about being undressed, but part of me knew it was wrong. She was older—probably fourteen or fifteen—and I did what she asked with trust. She was the first person I ever met who had a mental disability, so I thought it was a normal thing for someone with a disability to do. I blocked out whether she molested me or not, but I remember her smiling and making our secret tryst a game. This was my introduction to sex, or at least to acts of a sexual nature.

As if those two issues weren't difficult enough for a young child to handle, a third situation arose. To this point, I'd been apathetic when it came to learning about my physical condition. I knew nothing about cystic fibrosis and that was okay with me. Okay, that is, until the night I opened an encyclopedia.

Chapter 3
The Enemy Exposed

The tension in my family about cystic fibrosis came to a head when I was about nine. It was a normal Friday night, except I'd procrastinated on a book report that was due on Monday. I had to write a report on Christopher Columbus. I hated book reports because they always seemed to get in the way of *Diff'rent Strokes*. I wanted an easy way out, so I asked my father who Christopher Columbus was. He looked disappointed, then said he wasn't going to help me.

"That's why I bought the encyclopedias in the den," he said. "You know how to use them."

I trudged into the den, pulled Volume C from the shelf, and began turning pages. Before I found Columbus though, I saw the entry for "cystic fibrosis." I shouldn't have been surprised to find it there (hey, it was an encyclopedia), but I was. My parents had always censored what I read and watched to limit what I knew about CF. Doctors gave us videotapes about cystic fibrosis, but my mom never let me watch them. She said I didn't need to see them, though the doctors had made it clear they were for me, too. I was afraid to ask why. I didn't want to upset my mother, or maybe I just didn't want to know.

That night I began to read about cystic fibrosis. There wasn't a lot of information. I learned that CF affects the lungs and pancreas and makes mucus thicken. I skipped the long, boring medical words. Then my eye caught a sentence. After I read it, I wished I'd skipped it, too. It said: "Cystic fibrosis patients normally die before the age of twenty-five." I must have read that line ten times, hoping I'd read it wrong the first nine. So this was what my parents were hiding from me. The kids at school were right: I was going to be dead. I began to cry.

I went to the kitchen and tearfully asked my parents, "Am I going to die?"

"Where did you hear that?" my mom asked. She was caught noticeably off guard by my question. She probably suspected a kid at school had been taunting me, but this time my information came from the encyclopedia they'd bought and kept in our house—the encyclopedia I'd been told was always 100 percent accurate.

I can't imagine how my parents felt then. Not only did their son discover what they were hiding, but he now realized a disease that his parents had given him was going to take his life much too soon.

I nearly exploded from the anger I felt inside. I was enraged that my parents had kept this from me. "I hate you!" I told them. "I wish I was dead!" I didn't really hate my parents and I didn't wish I was dead, but I wanted to make a point. If I hated anything, it was cystic fibrosis, the disease that robbed me of a normal childhood.

Mom began to cry, but said quite firmly, "You are not going to die."

"Then why are you crying?" I screamed. "I hate you."

When my mother ran upstairs, I was stunned. I'd never spoken to her so viciously before. My father got angry with me, and told me to apologize to my mother.

"Apologize for what?" I demanded. "The fact that I am going to die?"

I realize now that I was being overly dramatic, but as a nine-year-old, I could not control my anger. I'd been beaten by a babysitter, thrown into a sexual tryst by a family friend, and now I'd learned I had a terminal disease and that my parents had been hiding it from me. I, too, ran upstairs to my room. I sat in the dark, pulled my royal blue Superman blanket over my head and cried. I kept thinking about the article in the encyclopedia. The facts were right there in black and white. My parents had lied to me, putting on happy faces and getting me to think I could lead a normal life. That was obviously not true. How could I ever trust them again? I realized then that I was absolutely terrified of death—mostly because I'd never faced it before. All of my grandparents were alive. No one I knew had passed away, and my sister Wendy had died before I was born, so I never knew her.

Eventually, my sobs quieted and I overheard my parents discussing the situation. I couldn't hear their words, but my father's tone was one of anger and disgust, and my mother sounded defensive.

That night might have been the first time I had the dream. I'm hiding under a clothes rack in a shopping mall when a brown-haired girl around my age finds me. She asks if I need help. I decline, thinking I could get myself out of this scary situation. She turns around, walks towards the exit and vanishes.

I didn't figure out until years later that the girl was Wendy. It was not a coincidence that the only times I had the dream were when cystic fibrosis reared its ugly head. As the only other member of my family who had CF, she was the one to whom I could truly relate. I firmly believe the dream was my sister's attempt to help me escape the anxiety that cystic fibrosis brought to my life. I only wished that she were alive then so I could have someone to talk to about the things that were happening to me—some of which I could never share with my parents.

The dream recurred many times over many years. I continued to be stubborn, though, and each time Wendy asked if I needed help, I refused. The truth was that I did need someone to step up, but to expect a nine-year-old child to recognize this was ridiculous. That's when someone else stepped in.

Chapter 4

My Father, My Hero

Early the next morning I awoke to a familiar voice.

"Get dressed," my father said. "We're going."

"No, I'm tired," I said from my bed, barely opening my eyes. "Leave me alone."

"Andy, get your butt out of bed," he said in a voice that meant business. "We're leaving."

I thought he might be throwing me out of the house for making my mom so upset and I felt a twinge of panic about where I would live.

"Where are we going?" I asked nervously. It was Saturday morning and I was eager for the lineup of my favorite cartoons. *Super Friends, The Flintstones, The Smurfs, Tom and Jerry,* and the *Looney Tunes* were all waiting for me. My morning was spoken for—if he let me stay.

"Baseball tryouts," my dad said. "It's time you went outside and learned to play sports. You'll thank me one day."

I panicked. Who was he kidding? The only thing I knew about sports was that I couldn't play them. I had been ridiculed in gym class more times than I cared to remember. I had no strength or stamina. Why didn't my father just accept that? As much as he wanted me to be like other sons, I wasn't.

"I don't want to go," I said, suddenly awake. "I can't play sports! Mom!"

Dad was unmoved. "Let's go," he said, pulling back the covers and tugging me out of bed.

I thought my mom would try to talk him out of this crazy scheme, but she didn't say anything. The woman who'd written dozens of notes to excuse me from gym class was silent. Maybe she was still mad at me. Maybe she wanted me to die.

Our first stop was the mall, where my dad had me try on countless baseball gloves until I found a comfortable one. Dad must really have been frustrated with me if he went to the mall. Even my mom couldn't drag him there. Next we drove to the field. It was dazzling green and there were lots of other boys with their parents. The coach told us to form lines so he could watch us run, catch, throw and hit. It sounded like gym class to me, and that didn't sound good.

23

I was by far the slowest, most awkward kid on the field. When a ball came toward me, I ducked. I wasn't sure which hand to wear my glove on. The coaches yelled at me, and the other kids laughed. I swung wildly at balls, but didn't hit a thing. As the humiliations mounted, I kept glancing at my dad for a sign that he'd seen enough and we could go home. But instead of the sign I was looking for, he told me to stay out there. Whenever I swung the bat, he'd offer the same advice: "Keep your eye on the ball." I wasn't sure what that meant.

After ninety minutes that felt like an eternity, tryouts were over. I dragged myself to the car and didn't say a word all the way home. What was there to say? That I let my dad down once again? That he'd finally seen proof that I was as uncoordinated a son as any man could have? I knew I couldn't be good enough for him. I wished he weren't my dad. I was so frustrated. Defiantly, I crossed my arms, huddled against the car door and thought, "I don't care!"

But slowly it came to me that, yes, I did care. It mattered to me that I couldn't do something well, and I wanted to change that. Baseball was different from gym class. Gym was only about what my teachers and classmates thought. Baseball was about my dad—someone I looked to for approval and someone I loved—despite occasional spells of thinking the contrary. When I was on the baseball field that morning, my mom couldn't excuse me with a note. My father could have taken me home, but he watched me and wouldn't let me leave. Instead of feeling angry at him, I was disappointed and disgusted with myself. I was also furious with the kids who'd ridiculed me. I wanted to change the way things were. I just wasn't sure how.

For the first time in my life, I wanted to better myself. I didn't want to be the worst athlete anymore. I didn't want to accept last place or be the tenth man on the bench. That night, for the first time, I joined my dad in the den as he watched an Atlanta Braves game on TV. There were players doing the same maneuvers on the field that I'd tried that day. They made the way they snagged a soaring ball in their glove or sent a ball sailing deep into the outfield look graceful and easy. My dad smiled as he watched them. I wanted him to smile like that when he saw me on the field. It was obvious I had a long way to go.

That night I couldn't sleep. After my parents went to bed, I grabbed my new mitt and a tennis ball and snuck into the basement. It was a spooky place, a dark unfinished room with shadowy corners that hid crickets, spider webs, and I didn't know what else. I made Howard come with me . . . just in case.

I wanted to show the guys on the field that I could play just as well as they did. No, not just as well—better. I wanted to earn their respect, in addition to my father's. I knew that wouldn't be easy. I threw the ball against the basement wall and tried to catch it the way the Major League players did. I missed. I dived, jumped and ran for the ball. I missed again and again. I felt more and more frustrated as I envisioned the entire Little League crowd laughing at me. I threw the ball about two hundred times before sneaking back to bed.

The next night I did the same thing. I had scraped-up knees and bruised shins, and sometimes I cut my elbows diving for balls. But I wouldn't let myself leave until I caught the ball and threw it a little better.

I'd like to say all that determination paid off. Truthfully, though, I was still the worst player on my team. Granted, I didn't duck anymore when a ball sailed in my direction, but I usually couldn't catch it either. When I was at bat, I didn't just hold the bat and wait for the ball to hit it. I actually swung. Not that I got any hits, but I was getting the hang of the game. I was still the last one picked for anything, but I was getting better.

Slowly, I was becoming a fixture in after-school neighborhood baseball games. Most of those games took place in our front yard with four or five players. The "field" was much smaller than a regulation baseball diamond. First base was the sewer that faced the street. Second and third base were the two weeping willows in front of our courtyard, and home plate was on our driveway. We used a tennis ball instead of a baseball and instead of tagging the base or the runner, all we had to do was peg the base runner with the ball below the waist and he was out. Anytime I came to the plate, my dog Howard—my biggest fan—barked from the courtyard, which I considered to be our dugout. I wasn't one of the better players, but I was getting outside, getting exercise, and meeting more people. I knew that pleased my dad.

The next season, I played with a team called the Knights. Maybe the word "played" is a bad choice. I was benched most of the season. I continued throwing the tennis ball against the basement wall at night and eventually exchanged the tennis ball for a blue racquetball. The racquetball came back faster and had a lot more jump. I continued to find good competition in our neighborhood scrimmages. I was making more plays, but I didn't know if that would translate to the field. During our Little League weekly practices, however, I could definitely see myself improving.

One fall night at practice, with my mom watching, I caught a fly ball in the outfield. Granted, I dropped seven others that night, but I caught one. I caught a ball! Unfortunately, my feat was lost in the fact that five minutes later our best hitter smashed a baseball over the fence that shattered a windshield.

My father was often busy with work, but sometimes I'd play catch with him. He would hit one towering fly ball after another until I caught one. He'd say, "You'll never get this one!" That would make me try even harder. We also regularly watched Braves games together and cheered on our team. That was the most fun I ever had with my dad. It was my way of showing him that I wanted to please him. Baseball became my way of telling my dad he could be proud of me. My first two seasons in Little League I knew I was no All-Star, but I vowed that the next year would be different.

The next spring when my Little League team, the Zephyrs, ran onto the field for opening day, I prayed I'd have a better season than I had with the Yankees and Knights. That wouldn't have taken much. I hadn't seen third base at all. Heck, second could have been a mirage for all I knew. So it was ironic that the coach positioned me at second base.

I glanced into the stands and found my parents among the crowd of chatting moms and dads. I didn't want to embarrass them. Instead, I wanted my dad to say proudly, "See the second baseman? That's my son, Andy." I hoped to show him how much I'd improved and how far I'd come as an athlete.

I was older than most of my teammates. Most of my Knights teammates had moved up to another division, but I was held back because I needed another year of seasoning at the tee league level. The first batter positioned himself by the tee, which the coaches always used for the first game of the season. He took a few practice swings and I grew increasingly edgy. Finally, he swung the bat, which made an extremely loud crack as it connected solidly with the ball. I noticed with a mix of excitement and fear that that very same ball was headed straight for me.

I leaped as high as my ten-year-old body could lift me and raised my gloved hand to meet the ball. When my feet hit the ground, I noticed the crowd was silent. The batter had stopped running toward first base. "Great," I thought. "I'm so bad that the runner actually had to stop to laugh."

Then I gazed into my glove, which to this point had been used mainly as a wig for the pumpkin lady my mom and I made on Halloween. Nestled inside was a round white object with red stitching. The baseball was in my possession, which could only mean I'd finally caught a ball in a real game. All those rigorous practices, scraped knees, bruised elbows and carpet burns had finally paid off. No longer would I be ridiculed for my poor play.

But the best memory of the day came a second later. I looked toward the stands and saw one man stand up and applaud as loudly and as enthusiastically as he would have if his kid had hit a home run with the bases loaded in the bottom of the ninth with the score tied to win the World Series. He hollered "All right, Andy!" so loudly that I had no trouble hearing him on the field. My dad was so proud of me that he proclaimed to everyone that I was his son! That day remains one of the most thrilling of my life.

Slowly, I was building the confidence that cystic fibrosis had been tearing down. And I was changing my relationship with my dad. I realized that the reason he'd sent me to Little League tryouts two seasons before was not to humiliate me. Instead, he wanted to show me that if I worked hard I could play well, just like anyone else. He didn't want me to use CF as an excuse for not trying or not excelling. Not in my wildest dreams did I ever think my father would be the one to help me. I loved him very much, but I always felt I could never meet his high expectations. Maybe the truth was that he had such high expectations because he saw potential in me.

With my baseball success, came an increased interest in watching sports on television. My room became a shrine with pictures of all my athlete idols—from Dale Murphy to Herschel Walker—cut from my *Sports Illustrated* magazines and tacked up on my bulletin board.

The Cystic Fibrosis Foundation found out about my newfound love of sports and gave me the chance to be a ball boy for the Atlanta Hawks, Atlanta's professional basketball team. The honor was a thank you for all the work my parents had done for the foundation. During pre-game warm-ups, I got to throw the ball to future Celtics Hall of Famers Larry Bird, Kevin McHale and Robert Parrish, who were playing the Hawks that night. The experience was awesome, but nothing like the second opportunity the Cystic Fibrosis Foundation gave me.

I became a sports fanatic the day my dad introduced me to the Atlanta Braves, and they became the way I determined how my day was going to go. If they won the night before, I had a little hop in my step. On days they lost, I analyzed every mistake and what moves Joe Torre, the Braves manager, should or should not have made. So when I found out that the Cystic Fibrosis Foundation granted my wish to be an honorary Braves batboy for a day, my face lit up. I was so excited to meet my baseball hero, Dale Murphy. It turned out he was one of the nicest guys I'd ever meet. He was very genuine and welcomed me to the dugout, and we even talked a little baseball before he signed some pictures for me. I got to meet several other Braves, too, including Glenn Hubbard, Willie Stargell and Bruce Benedict. During my day as batboy I brought balls to the umpires and picked up bats after the players dropped them. I loved every second of it. Two highlights of the game, which the Braves won 8-6, were a three-run go-ahead home run from Murphy, and a fifth inning brawl in which Bill Gullickson, a Reds pitcher, plunked one of the Braves in the back. All the players ran out of the dugout and I grabbed a bat and pretended I was getting involved so my parents could snap a picture. That afternoon at Atlanta's Fulton County Stadium stands out in my mind as the greatest sports moment of my youth.

The Braves did another important thing for me—something even more significant than letting me be a batboy for a day. The Braves brought my father and me together. My dad loved *60 Minutes* and other news shows, and I loved cartoons, but we could not stand to watch each other's programs. The Braves games were the only thing we watched together. My father and I sat on the couch in the den and focused on the team wearing red, white and blue. On occasion, we visited Fulton County Stadium, where we sat in the upper deck, prayed for a foul ball and watched our favorite team battle their opponents. It was nice that for once the focal point between us was something other than cystic fibrosis.

My newfound interest in baseball showed me that sports could not only serve as a distraction from CF and the other horror stories of my childhood, but also as a reminder that hard work and determination could lead to success. That lesson was also vividly evident on the tennis court.

Chapter 5
Finding Fire Through Sports

"I take Brian."

"I take Josh."

"I take Keith."

"I take Kristie."

"I take Dina."

And after everyone else was picked, "I guess we'll take Andy."

That was how every physical education class went for me from first to fourth grade. I dreaded those days when my classmates chose teams because I was almost always the last pick. I had low self-esteem to begin with and didn't need the constant five-day-a-week reminder in the gymnasium.

But as I got more involved in sports, I noticed something. I was doing a lot better in my fifth grade gym class. Finally, I was actually finishing the laps. I didn't have to quit. The teacher did not have to blow the whistle so that I'd stop walking. Then something even more remarkable happened. One by one, kids were finishing after me. First it was the girls. Then slowly I started finishing ahead of some of the guys. Then I started finishing ahead of most of the guys. I wasn't last anymore. I didn't need any more notes from my mom. I was doing something relatively amazing for someone with CF. I was fitting in.

By the end of fifth grade, I had won the award for most improved athlete! It was not honor roll or super honor roll, but this award, for me, was even bigger. I'd learned earlier that year that I was not supposed to be alive at twenty-five, and that I shouldn't be able to do lots of things normal kids do. That award alleviated a lot of my doubts. Sports absolutely showed me the way.

When I was ten, my dad introduced me to tennis. I was good at baseball, but I certainly was never going to get All-Star consideration or be an MVP. I was a below average basketball player, an even worse soccer player and I was lucky I didn't drown as a swimmer . . . but, there was something about tennis.

My friend and classmate, Josh Yudin, and I started taking group tennis lessons. I found I enjoyed tennis and began practicing every day, hitting the ball with my father, my mother, Aunt Susie and Uncle Bobby. Before I knew it, my mom enrolled me at the Atlanta Jewish Community Center's tennis camp.

After a few clinics, I felt I was improving, but was disappointed to learn the instructors felt differently. We were being grouped by skill and I was assigned to the lowest level while all my friends, including Josh, were in the highest level. Practicing with the kids in my group, I got really tired of going into the woods every five minutes to retrieve tennis balls. I hadn't seen that many balls sail over a fence since I watched highlights of baseball great Hank Aaron's career. Still, I kept practicing with my aunt and uncle and both my parents.

Just before camp ended, our instructor announced that we'd play a round-robin tournament. The champion at each level would receive a trophy. As soon as she said the word "trophy," I knew I wanted it. Our instructor needed a fourth person for the round robin in the high level tournament and had finally seen some improvement in my game, so she chose me. I'm sure she thought I would be an easy win for my three opponents, but I really wanted a chance to play against my friends, instead of the kids on the lower level.

That night, I repeatedly tossed a tennis ball against the living room wall to prepare for the upcoming baseball season. I had moved my practice field upstairs after I found a baby snake in the basement. My mom had told me a zillion times not to play ball in the living room—isn't that a standard Momism?—but, of course, I didn't listen. I had developed a pretty accurate arm and hadn't broken any of her good china or knickknacks. Yet.

My toss was about three inches to the right, and the ball sailed into a vase, knocking it onto the tile floor. It shattered. I couldn't believe it. What was I going to tell my mom?

There was nothing to say, because as soon as she saw that her favorite vase was missing, she knew what had happened. She yelled at me and sent me to bed with no television. I cried, hoping to make her feel guilty, but she knew that trick. The next morning she told me how disappointed she was.

"Fine," I sulked. "Punish me. I won't play in the tennis tournament. Are you happy now?"

She looked at me thoughtfully, and then said something I'll never forget. "You'd better play, because you are going to win and put the trophy where the vase used to be." Then she grinned and gave me a hug.

The day of the tournament, I was infused with motivation. I was going to return home with a trophy and put a smile on my mom's face. My first opponent was Graham Stieglitz, one of my close friends.

When camp started, Graham and I had pretty equal skills, but I'd definitely gotten better while we were there. My main weapon was consistency, something Graham did not possess. I won four of the five games we played.

Next, I faced Adam Strohl, the prior year's tournament winner and an undefeated player at camp. I'd lost to him five times already and had only just racked up my first win against Graham. I was nervous. Adam was the John McEnroe of our tournament. He wasn't just supposed to win; he was supposed to cruise. But something peculiar happened in that first game: I won. I'm still not sure how. After that, the butterflies left my stomach and confidence flowed into my head. I remembered that my mother wanted me to win the trophy, and I wanted to win it for her. I wasn't leaving without it. We finished our set. Adam won three games. I won five.

My last competitor was Josh, whom I'd never beaten. He hadn't seen my match against Adam and asked how I did. When I told him I'd beaten Adam, his eyes widened.

"Are you kidding?" he said.

I told him I'd played the best I ever had. That, of course, motivated Josh to want to beat me. I was the last of the undefeated players. We ended up splitting our match three games each. I'd never beaten Josh before, so that was a moral victory.

Tired and sweaty, we gathered around our instructor. And Adam's dad, one of the camp volunteers, punched our results into his calculator. The trophy would go to whoever won the highest percentage of games. The drizzle that was falling while I was playing Adam had become a light shower. Judging from the dark clouds overhead, it was getting ready to pour. I was so nervous that my hands were shaking and my stomach ached. The rain began to fall faster. Finally, Adam's dad was finished.

"Adam won a total of 13 of 21 games," he said, "and Andy won 12 of 19."

Darn. I lost by a game. That's not fair; I beat him. My mom gave me a hug, but I pushed her away. "Why are you hugging me?" I said. "I lost."

"No, you didn't," she said.

Adam's father continued: "That means Andy won 63 percent of his games, and Adam won 62 percent. Congratulations, Andy."

Oh, my gosh! I won. I couldn't believe it when I was handed the most beautiful trophy I'd ever seen. Sure, it was plastic and the inscription was a little blurry, but it was mine. I had earned it, and it was especially meaningful because it was my first individual accomplishment ever. The rain was pouring now, and Mom and I ran to the car. Fortunately for me, a plastic trophy isn't likely to warp or tarnish. I told her we could put it on the table where the vase used to stand, and she smiled.

That trophy gave me the confidence to venture into other sports. I started playing basketball. In fact, my basketball goal became the neighborhood hotspot and soon I was playing four or five pickup games a day with some older kids on the block. With the frequent baseball scrimmages still taking place in our front yard, I was becoming a regular sports participant. That's not to say I was the world's best athlete. There were a lot of kids better than I, but it was difficult to find someone who enjoyed playing sports more.

Tennis made me a fiery competitor. When I won matches, I would dissect every game afterward and identify the key points of the match. When I lost, I took it hard. I'd criticize myself endlessly and force myself to practice even more. Uncle Bobby taped me practicing and we would go to his house and examine every little mistake I made. It sounds obsessive, but it was good for me. It gave me a strong work ethic—something I would need to beat cystic fibrosis.

I often wonder what would have happened had I not won the round robin. Would I have blamed cystic fibrosis and gone back into my shell? Did one percentage point change the way I believed in myself? Did one tennis round robin change who I was?

Eventually, I accumulated a collection of about thirty trophies, but none more important than the one I won for my mom that rainy afternoon. That day, I was better than anyone on the tennis court. It didn't matter that I had cystic fibrosis. What mattered was that I had faith in myself and that I worked hard. From time to time, I still look at that trophy. It's only six inches high and it doesn't even have my name on it. It's more than just a plastic memento, though. It's a reminder that someone who wasn't given much of a chance triumphed because of perseverance, practice and support. It didn't matter that I was only ten years old and that it was just a tennis round robin. I viewed it as a sign that by working hard and not giving up, beating something like cystic fibrosis was possible. That is the lesson I learned, and it is a lesson so important that it has kept me alive.

Chapter 6
Man's Best Friend

My earliest memory of Howard is a bundle of brown fur attached to a tail that wagged faster than Carl Lewis ran. Howard zoomed into my life when I was four, and Aunt Anita and Uncle Jerry, along with my parents, conspired to surprise me with a pet.

Our meeting got off to what you might call a bad start. I was so excited to have a dog that I darted after this puppy, who was not quite as excited about having a four-year-old buddy and an unfamiliar home. He promptly bit me on the hand. It served me right. We made up minutes later, though, and we were inseparable after that. I don't know who was more thrilled to have a playmate, Howard or me.

Howard grew into a loveable mutt who weighed about thirty-five pounds. My Aunt Susie called him a true Heinz 57 because no one really knew what breed he was. His father, Hunky, was my Aunt Anita's dog and Hunky was a mutt, too. Howard had long brown hair, a sweet face, and for many years was my best friend.

When I was sick and other kids were playing baseball or tag in our yard, I watched from inside, peering through the glass door in the den and wishing I could be outside with them. Howard always kept me company. He'd put his head in my lap, and I swear he knew how depressed I was. His ears were the only ones I confessed my secrets to. He was the only one who knew about the family friend. He was the only one who knew how much I feared the babysitter and how scared I was to die.

Because I couldn't run around a lot, I loved to watch him lope through the yard, ears flapping and fur shining. I felt he was an emissary for me, that because I couldn't run, he was doing it for me.

If Howard was smart, he hid it well. He didn't know a single trick. When I told him to sit, he would lie down. When I told him to roll over, he would lie down. When I told him to shake, well, you get the idea. He was a great garbage disposal, though. That poor dog ate many pounds of spinach, discreetly ferried from my plate to his mouth whenever my mom turned her head during dinner. I still owe him for that. What a pal.

As much as I loved him, Howard was a crazy dog. Sometimes he'd leave for days at a time and then come back with a look that said he did something very wrong. He was the gigolo of the neighborhood . . . we guessed this after seeing many different litters of Howard-like puppies. He chased fire trucks, played in our messy creek and ran after any animal that was smaller than he was. He wasn't aggressive, just overly playful; he had a lot of energy. That is until the day he ran onto someone else's property behind our backyard woods and a loud bang echoed through the trees. Howard had been shot in the leg.

We never found the person who shot him, but after the gunshot, Howard had a severe limp. That wasn't the worst, though. A few years later, he came home whimpering. I thought maybe he hurt his leg again, so I rubbed it. He didn't react much, but when I petted him, he yelped in pain. Mom and I quickly discovered twenty bees stuck to his collar, stinging him. We ripped the collar off and some of the bees began flying around our house. Howard licked us in appreciation. It was around that time we decided to have him neutered. He lost a little of his energy and couldn't escape the wall of our courtyard anymore, but Howard still had that sense of timing when I needed him and one day I certainly did.

One afternoon I was tossing my green Nerf football to myself. In my mind, I could hear the cheers of a stadium full of fans, wild with glee that I'd snared the touchdown pass to end the tie and win the game. The crowd went crazy as I waved nonchalantly. Just another stellar Lipman performance on the gridiron. The sound was deafening.

Wait. It wasn't the sound that was deafening. It was the silence. The afternoon had become eerily still with the exception of the sound of something approaching on four feet, something that sounded like a dog, but it wasn't Howard. It was Max. I knew it before I even saw him.

Every kid in my neighborhood—and even some adults—was terrified of this black Doberman. He had killed two other dogs and sent a boy to the hospital. At least that was the rumor. I didn't see any reason not to believe it. Max looked anything but friendly. My parents had warned me more than once to stay away from him. Not that I needed any caution.

I hadn't gone looking for him, yet here he was in my yard, rapidly advancing on me with his tongue hanging from between rows of sharp teeth and an evil look in his eye. The sound of his chained collar could not be mistaken. Who knows what he was thinking? Maybe he saw the football and wanted to play? Maybe he was just curious? I didn't really want to find out. As he advanced, I felt exactly the way a wide receiver looks before a defensive back slams him to the ground. Then I began to run. But a ten-year-old with CF is no match for a full-grown Doberman.

Suddenly, Max was on top of me, panting and pawing. I tried to push him away, but that just seemed to make him more aggressive. He bit my leg just below my shorts. I began to cry in panic. Where was everyone? Where was my mom? Would Max carry me off after he'd killed me, or would he tear off my leg and leave me to bleed to death? What if my mother found my bloody body in the back yard? I gasped and tried to scream, but my voice was clenched inside me.

Suddenly, I heard a ringing sound. It was the sound of a dog tag clanking against a collar. It was the familiar sound that Howard made wherever he went, and he was racing for Max and me. He must have known I was in serious trouble because he lunged for the Doberman and sunk his teeth into the dog. Max yowled in pain, but Howard held on. Now Max was really mad. I was terrified because Max had already killed two other dogs. What if Howard was next? I wanted to help him fight Max, but I was so terror-stricken that I couldn't get up.

Run, run, Howard, I willed, trying to communicate with him with my mind, the way I often did. Run! Run! Howard either didn't hear me or wasn't listening. He and Max were wrestling furiously on the grass. They were just a swirl of fur and teeth. Then, I heard the loudest scream I've ever heard from a dog. Until that moment, I didn't know dogs were capable of screaming. It was an eerie, high-pitched sound, almost like a horn or an air-raid siren. If I were a dog, I would've been terrified.

A dog wrenched himself from the tussle and began limping away. Howard? No, it was Max. To my astonishment Howard, who was twenty pounds lighter, was chasing Max. Max kept looking back to see Howard right behind him and both disappeared behind the courtyard and into the woods. What if Max turned and began chasing Howard? I found my voice and screamed, "Come back! Howard! Come back!"

I'm not sure how long I waited. I'm not sure if I thought Howard would come back. But he did. I can't say he looked smug, though he did have the air of someone who's finished a rather annoying chore and is ready to move on to something more enjoyable. He was panting and there were spots of blood on his leg.

Max was nowhere in sight. In fact, he never returned to our neighborhood again. Howard, who didn't know a single trick, knew how to make Max disappear. I don't know what happened to Max, but I'd like to think he crawled off into the woods and died, the one and only victim of the gentlest, sweetest dog in the world.

Howard sat with me on the grass until I felt sturdy enough to make my way inside. My mom hadn't heard any of the commotion, so I showed her the puncture wounds on my leg and babbled about Howard's bravery and courage. Without a second thought, he risked his life for me, and I honestly believe he saved my life.

I think of cystic fibrosis as having some of the same menacing and terrifying qualities that Max did, though without that nasty dog breath, and I think of Howard as embodying the most productive attitude to have about CF. Though he knew his opponent was bigger and had defeated others, he fearlessly confronted it, and through his determination, chased it off. Undaunted, Howard basically said, "Never give up." Without saying a word, he set an amazing example.

Every April 1st, when I was a kid, I celebrated Howard's birthday by giving him a burger with a candle in it. I didn't know if his birthday really was April 1st, but considering his inability to perform any tricks whatsoever, a birthday on April Fools' Day seemed to make sense.

Friends came and went, but Howard was a loyal constant. His love never changed, and he couldn't have cared less whether I made a team or was cut, whether I was bent over, red-faced and heaving from coughing spells or whether I slumped through a day feeling like the biggest loser in the world. To Howard, I was a best friend—exactly what he was to me.

Chapter 7
The Best and Worst of Being Twelve

I was an only child for most of my younger years and didn't understand why my parents didn't have other kids. All of my close friends had siblings. I didn't realize my parents had given up on having children because Wendy and I both were born with CF. My parents recognized that another child with cystic fibrosis would not only have a difficult life, but could also give and get infections from me. In retrospect, this meant that, had Wendy lived, I probably never would have existed.

On September 4, 1985—my twelfth birthday—my parents had a wish come true. Unbeknownst to me, they had filed adoption papers and I was soon going to have a sibling. I remember their joy the night I heard them tell Aunt Susie and Uncle Bobby about the new baby. I felt so left out. This was my birthday and everyone was talking about another child.

Emily Robyn Lipman was born less than two months later, and while I was jealous, initially, I quickly grew to love her as much as my parents did. Emily grew up like most children. She had lots of toys, several pets and plenty of friends. However, unlike most children she had an older brother with a life-threatening disease.

When Emily was very young, I taught her how to take pills. She was afraid to take them and my mom had no luck teaching her. One day, I said, "Look at me. I take thirty to forty pills a day. And you can't take one?" That afternoon my sister learned to take pills.

Em became used to my therapy when she was still a baby. I let her sit near me while the vest vibrated and we watched cartoons or played video games. There was an obvious age difference. While I was in high school, she was still in preschool. And while I was applying for colleges, she was finger painting. I had fun with Emily, though, and taught her about the things I loved and wanted her to love, too. We played basketball on the driveway. I taught her how to use a bat and hit the tennis ball over the neighbor's yard for a home run. I showed her how watching a horror movie with no sound actually made it a comedy.

Most importantly, I taught Emily that life was worth living.

·····

Most nights my parents watched TV at night before going to bed. Well, I shouldn't say "watched" because usually the TV was background noise while they talked to each other or chatted on the phone. After finishing my homework, I'd often join them and watch the conclusion of whatever show they were watching, or, more often, weren't watching.

One night, I noticed something unusual before I entered their bedroom. Standing in the doorway, I could see them both focused intently on the screen. That was odd. If what they were watching was so good, why hadn't they called me so I could see it, too?

I held very still, trying to figure out what was going on and hoping that my parents wouldn't notice me. I spotted something peculiar on the bed—a box of tissues nestled between my parents. At the commercial break, my mom grabbed a tissue, wiped her eyes and blew her nose. There was already a little pile of wadded-up tissues on the night table by her side of the bed. I wondered what the heck was happening.

When the show resumed, I snuck a glance at the screen and saw something I'd never seen before—a girl using the same type of aerosol therapy that I used. She was also getting the same type of chest-thumping therapy my parents gave me. It was about time, I thought. Finally, I'd seen someone who knew what my life was like. She looked like a really nice girl, too—someone I could be friends with, maybe. She reminded me of Wendy, who frequented my dreams back then. Then I saw something that completely disrupted my thinking. Doubled over in pain, this adorable little girl began to cough up blood, gasp and cry out in pain.

At that moment my mother saw me. "Go to your room and go to bed!" she yelled. "You don't need to be watching this."

That was exactly what I needed to hear. Anything that I shouldn't be watching was something I didn't want to miss, especially if it involved someone with CF.

"But I want to watch it," I pleaded.

"Go to bed!" she repeated. It was clear that arguing wasn't an option.

I had another plan, though. I obediently went into my room and shut the door. But instead of going to bed, I switched on the television in my bedroom and turned down the volume so my parents wouldn't hear the sound. There was the girl, this time looking very frail, lying in bed, her parents at her side. They were sobbing.

Before I could catch up with the story, in stormed my mother. She was still crying, and her mascara made gray smears down her face. She clicked off the TV and ordered me into bed. It was clear that she did not want me to watch whatever tragic story was being played out on TV.

The next morning everything was "normal." We didn't talk about the show or what happened to the girl or why my parents were crying. But I wasn't stupid. I began to worry that, like the girl in the movie, I too would cough up blood and become bed-ridden. No one could live like that, so I knew I would die. Other questions raced through my twelve-year-old brain: Was there terrible pain for her? What had happened to her? Would the same thing happen to me?

My family tried everything in their power to keep me healthy so I wouldn't end up like the girl from the movie. My father kept pushing me to play sports. My mother kept me away from sick children in the neighborhood.

And my Uncle Bobby . . . well, he had a different plan.

Chapter 8
Running on Empty

Every time my Uncle Bobby wore his Peachtree Road Race T-shirt, I swear my mouth watered. People saw him wearing it and had all kinds of questions: "Bobby, how long did you train?" "How did you do it?" "How many races have you run?" He'd always have a story about the smothering heat on race day or his fellow runners or the exhaustion he faced as he neared the finish line. Hearing him talk, I always wished I could be the one telling those stories.

"The Peachtree," as it's called, is the biggest 10K race in the world. It brings tens of thousands of runners to Atlanta each July 4th. Police close off 6.2 miles of road and runners take over. Thousands of cheering fans line the streets with homemade signs of encouragement and cups of water for the runners. Many runners are professionals from around the world who whip across the finish line with astounding times, but most are people who can be seen every day running through neighborhoods—joggers and runners who've set their sights on a goal and move toward it.

Everyone who crosses the finish line receives a Peachtree Road Race T-shirt. These shirts are not available for sale, and no runner who finished the race in the extreme Georgia heat would ever give his away. The only way to get one is to run the entire race.

Uncle Bobby had about nine Peachtree T-shirts, which was no surprise. He had been a football coach and had run in the Boston and New York marathons. He was very big on motivation. If you weren't motivated, you couldn't earn his respect. Though he was married to my Aunt Susie, I didn't really like Bobby much because he was so tough on me.

Other relatives, knowing I had CF, sometimes coddled me, but Bobby would have none of that. My father and I would play my aunt and uncle in doubles, and they'd always win. The two of them combined had more trophies than I had excuses. I was envious of the easy grace Bobby had on the court. He didn't have to work as hard as I did, yet he continued to whip my butt.

It really irked me that I couldn't beat him, and he certainly wasn't going to throw a game my way out of sympathy. With Bobby, if you were going to win, you had to earn it. That made me resent him, but it also grudgingly earned my lasting respect. More than ever, I wanted to beat him because in some way it would be like beating CF.

True to his nature as a coach, Bobby was glad to help me shape up, though he often did it with sarcasm. He'd built up a big lead and then launch into, "Your mama's so fat. . ." jokes just to deepen the insult. But, hey, it worked. Bobby helped me train nearly every day when I was a fifth grader and, as a result, I won the most improved athlete award that year. Most people wouldn't remember that award, but to me it was very important that I could finally compete with my classmates, instead of handing the teacher an excuse.

Yet it wasn't enough. I still couldn't beat Bobby, so I decided to join him. I wanted to earn a Peachtree T-shirt, and I knew that, despite the taunts, Bobby would be the best person to train and motivate me.

We began when I was thirteen with two or three miles at a time, twice a week. It took nearly six months to build up to five miles. It helped that we trained along the actual race route, Peachtree Road, Atlanta's most famous street. Every night after training, I went to sleep thinking how good it would feel to wear the race T-shirt that I was going to earn.

One day, less than two weeks before the race, I ran five miles and then played tennis with Josh for an hour and a half. When I stretched to hit a ball, I felt a weird twinge in my right ankle. It didn't hurt, really, so I kept playing, but later that night, it still felt strange. The next morning I couldn't walk without limping. It wasn't as if I needed crutches; it was just an awkward feeling in my ankle. I refused to see a doctor, but decided I'd best take the day off from running.

I reluctantly told Bobby he'd have to train without me. He was disappointed because he never doubted I had the ability to run the race. He didn't want me to give up, but he also knew that I had to get to that point myself.

As each day passed, my confidence eroded a little more. Mentally, I could not get past the 6.2 miles with a potentially swollen ankle in the extreme summer heat. I'd run up to five miles, but I'd never done it with thousands of runners beside me. I'd never done it on a humid July day. I'd never hit 6.2 miles. My confidence was completely gone when, a week before the race I lost my number, my ticket to the Peachtree. My parents sold it out from under me to a runner who hadn't gotten one of the coveted numbers. Because the race is so popular, there aren't enough spaces for everyone who wants to run, so there's a big demand for numbers. People can and do actually buy numbers from people who aren't running.

As soon as this woman happily handed her fifteen dollars to my parents, I realized my dream of running that year's Peachtree was truly gone. She smiled at me, grateful for a ticket to the race. I glared back stoically, in an effort to hide my disappointment.

"You should be ashamed," I thought, "for taking a kid's number. You took my T-shirt. You took my dream." Deep inside, though, I knew this runner was nothing more than a bystander in the internal battle I was constantly fighting with myself.

On the morning of July 4th, I watched the race on TV. I couldn't bear to join the crowd downtown that was urging on the runners. The cameras were fixed on the finish line, where runner after runner joyously pumped their arms into the air at the victory and the accomplishment. My ankle no longer hurt. Truth be told, I'm not sure it ever did. I'd let the Peachtree Road Race beat me that day, and because I had cystic fibrosis, the odds of me getting a second chance were slim.

Bobby called me that afternoon. "Have a good sleep?" he teased, knowing that if I'd been running the race, I would have been up before six A.M.

"Just fine," I said. "I don't care about some stupid race. I'll run it next year."

I didn't run the next year, though, or the year after, or the year after that. Instead, I concentrated on tennis. And when I was fourteen, I did the impossible. After hundreds of losses on the court, I defeated Uncle Bobby. With every point I won, I felt a changing of the guard. After all these years, I was the athlete in the family. Well, not quite. Bobby still had a whole drawer of Peachtree Road Race T-shirts. I had a drawer full of polo shirts. Uncle Bobby was just the type of person to remind me of that.

While I had other opportunities to train for the Peachtree, I was intimidated by the race. I feared it some days as much as CF. For years, so many people told me that I had limitations. Sure, I was playing baseball and tennis, but neither of those compared to running a ten-kilometer race. I kept thinking about the article I read that said I'd be dead at twenty-five. I thought about all the times my mom begged me not to over-exert myself. I thought about the doctors and the negative news that came with most appointments.

It was difficult not to lament over cystic fibrosis. Doctor visits were tough. We often visited Dr. Caplan at Grady Memorial Hospital, where an entire wing was dedicated to CF. At the time, there were no adult CF centers. Kids with CF were considered middle-aged. Half their lives were assumed to be over. The doctors were pessimistic about everyone.

As a child, having a life threatening disease made me a lot more mature than other kids. My biggest concern wasn't baseball card collecting or getting an "A" on a book report. My biggest concern was staying as healthy as possible. I didn't want to end up in the hospital.

Although I was doing far better than Dr. Caplan ever imagined, I usually got bad news at my appointments. Playing baseball and my brief attempts to run the Peachtree were helping my pulmonary numbers, yet I still coughed a lot. My medications seemed ineffective. My mom was frustrated.

One day on vacation in St. Augustine, Florida, Mom and Nana Rose were walking with me when I began to cough uncontrollably. I was scared. The movie about the girl with CF made me realize that things could get bad fast. My mom was at her wit's end. She and my dad began researching doctors outside Atlanta. My parents needed a miracle worker.

And finally, they found him.

Chapter 9
A Rescue Boat

By the time I turned fifteen, we had moved to nearby Dunwoody, Georgia. My parents had grown frustrated with the care I was getting and began going to the Emory University Medical Library to research doctors who specialized in cystic fibrosis. They called doctors around the country, including the Mayo Clinic in Rochester, Minnesota, but none made my parents feel comfortable that these doctors could help me. It was as if my parents were crazy for thinking a child with cystic fibrosis could live a better life.

My Aunt Loretta, who was my father's sister, had worked for the Cystic Fibrosis Foundation in Rhode Island and gave my parents the name of a doctor she'd heard good things about. My parents called and spoke to him for a very long time. They decided it was worth a drive to the University of North Carolina to meet him.

A few months later, my parents and I made the three hundred mile drive to Chapel Hill to meet the up-and-coming doctor. I honestly didn't believe there was a doctor anywhere who could help me. My life-long negative experiences with doctors made me believe that CF was invincible.

I was edgy the first time I visited the UNC Children's Hospital. Upon arriving, I was subjected to a parade of sick, dying and helpless children. Quite honestly, it terrified me. I saw a boy a few years younger than I in a wheelchair in a corner of the waiting room. His eyes, set deep in a pale face, were glassy and barely open. Tubes were connected to his frail arms. He coughed continuously and looked like he was in pain.

I was in the pulmonary department when I overheard someone say the little boy had cystic fibrosis. Reading about cystic fibrosis in an encyclopedia was one thing. Seeing a person suffering—someone with the same genetic disorder I had—well, that was another thing entirely. I could always close a book, but I couldn't close my eyes and ears to the person sitting across from me. I wondered how long he would live or if he even wanted to live. Then I asked the same questions about myself. How long did I have to live? Would I end up a shadow of myself, confined to a wheelchair, a burden on my parents and a pitiful sight to other people? That became my biggest fear.

45

That afternoon, a tall man with a dark beard and white hospital coat walked in and said, "Hello, Andy. How are you? I'm Tom Boat." Strangely, he seemed positive about my future. Even stranger was that I believed he meant it. Dr. Boat was a nice guy with a good sense of humor and, most importantly, one of the brightest CF doctors in the country. He had told my parents he could make enormous improvements in my health by treating me aggressively and changing my medical routine. He was way ahead of his time.

Dr. Boat then demonstrated the devices he used. They seemed a lot more advanced than the ones I'd seen at Grady. I had a lot of tests that day and, afterward, Dr. Boat adjusted most of my medications. From my pills to my aerosol treatments, Dr. Boat made the wholesale changes he promised. Dr. Boat's belief that he could make me stronger reminded me of the poster that had become my touchstone so many years ago. I thought of the muscular man with cystic fibrosis whose picture hung on the wall. I believed that, yes, I could be that guy.

Dr. Boat was also instrumental in my most significant lifestyle change to date. He helped find the bronchial therapy machine I got when I was about sixteen. My mom had to fight with the insurance company to get them to pay for it, but it was worth the hassle.

For some sixteen-year-olds, a car means freedom. For me, the chest therapy machine was the equivalent. It changed my life. Before I got the microwave-sized box, my parents had to do my chest therapy every day from the time I was two weeks old. Each morning I lay on a pillow and my father or mother cupped their hands and thumped all over my chest. It made a popping sound, and the process loosened the mucus in my lungs. Then I took three deep breaths, coughed up the phlegm and spit it into the toilet between position changes. I had to switch positions six times so they could cover my whole chest. The process was a huge hassle, but we did it every single day.

Therapy didn't really hurt, but it certainly wasn't fun, and it consumed nearly an hour every day. During therapy, I couldn't watch television, read or talk. I felt trapped. I know it was hard for my parents, too. They'd been administering therapy to me before I even knew why it was being done. When I was an infant and toddler, they had to hold me down while I screamed and struggled . . . and they could never take a day off.

I was always concerned that I'd never be able to leave home because I needed my parents to perform my therapy. As I went through high school and my friends began visiting colleges, this weighed on me more and more. I wanted to go to a university, too, but I sure as heck didn't want to take my parents with me. Commuting from home didn't really appeal to me because I wanted the "real" college experience of going to a new place and being on my own. I began to think that there was no point in making good grades. I wouldn't be able to attend college. I was going to be left behind.

Then the bronchial therapy machine came along. When I turned it on, the machine sounded like a vacuum cleaner. The loud noise made it difficult to watch television but I quickly became accustomed to lip-reading. Its vest fitted snugly around my chest and sent currents that vibrated my chest. I used six frequencies for five minutes each, while making the vest tighter or looser. The great thing about the machine was that I could do my aerosol therapy—the mist treatment that I inhaled through a nebulizer—at the same time, which shaved twenty-five minutes from my routine. I could play video games during the treatment, but reading was pretty much out of the question. The constant shaking of the vest caused the words to bounce around on the page. Still the positives far outweighed the negatives. Having the machine was incredibly freeing and made a huge lifestyle change, both for me and for my parents.

The therapy machine, while extremely heavy, was portable. It could be wheeled anywhere. That meant I could go on vacations and trips with friends without my parents tagging along. Eventually, the manufacturer redesigned the machine, making it much smaller, slightly quieter and even easier for travel.

That same year, an exciting development on the CF front was revealed. One night in the fall of 1989, my mom excitedly called upstairs. From her expression I knew something unusual was happening. "Andy, look!" she said motioning toward the TV. "Look what they're talking about." It was a news story announcing that the CF gene had been discovered.

"Will that cure me?" I asked. I believed this was the most she and I had conversed about cystic fibrosis since the day I was born.

"Not yet," she said, "but a cure is definitely within reach." For years, doctors had predicted a cure was expected in seven to ten years. I wondered if that were still the case. My mom's excitement got me thinking that maybe I didn't have to have cystic fibrosis anymore. Maybe this therapy machine was a short-term solution. Maybe I'd be cured. Maybe I'd live a normal life.

There was no cure in the immediate future, but the vest I'd gotten had changed my life. My health was getting better and I couldn't just credit that to the machine. Dr. Boat made a big difference in my life.

And so did Josh.

Chapter 10
My Partner in Crime

Batman had Robin. Starsky had Hutch. And in a small Atlanta suburb, Andy Lipman had Josh Yudin. My first memory of him is as a six-year-old kid my size with red hair and an attitude. We were going to be attending the same school, and our mothers had been put in touch so they could carpool. While they got acquainted in Josh's mom's kitchen, we watched TV for a few minutes and then got in a huge fight. Hair was pulled, punches were thrown. I cried all the way home. We've been friends ever since.

We learned tennis, basketball and baseball together. We weren't amazing athletes, but we were tough competitors and we had a lot of fun. In our first basketball league, the coach never let us have the ball, which really frustrated us. One day in practice, though, the coach passed it to me. Looking back, it might have been an accident. I turned to Josh and said, "You have to feel this thing. I knew it was round, but I didn't think it was so rough." We thought that was hysterical, but the coach didn't. He continued benching us.

Josh and I spent every waking hour together. We both performed in school talent shows, though neither of us had any identifiable talent. We both had a crush on our fourth-grade teacher, Ms. Powell. We spent so much time together that friends mixed us up. They'd call me Josh and him Andy. If they saw Josh, they'd ask where I was, and if they saw me, they'd ask where Josh was.

The only time we were rivals was in competition, unless, of course, we were playing doubles in tennis. Josh was the only guy I didn't beat when I won that trophy at tennis camp. We tied. In second grade he beat me in the finals of the school spelling bee. I will never misspell "invisible" again. But there was no shame in losing any academic competition to Josh. He was a very bright guy. By the time third grade rolled around, I knew there were three certainties in life: death, taxes, and Josh would be on the honor roll. Josh was in every advanced class while I was a mainstay in the general level classes. That didn't change our friendship, though. Josh and I kept each other in hysterics with different brands of humor. Josh's jokes were long stories. They took a while to develop; nonetheless, the punch line almost always delivered laughter from his audience. Mine were corny puns, the type of jokes that came in a Cracker Jack box.

A lot of people hung around Josh because he made them laugh, but that wasn't the reason he and I were such good friends. Josh and I were like brothers. Each of us had—and still has—a lot of respect for the other, but that never stopped us from wanting to beat the other's butt. The fierce competitiveness we shared only brought us closer. Josh once broke both his feet in a two-on-two basketball tournament, but he finished the game. That was stupid, but it demonstrated his toughness. He used to tell me, "If you try zero percent of the time, you'll fail 100 percent of the time."

Josh has never treated me differently because I have cystic fibrosis. When I coughed, he never asked if I was okay. When I gasped for air, he didn't pity me. On the contrary, he pushed me to work harder. If I was losing a tennis match or basketball game, he'd urge me to rally and win. That meant a lot to me, because when I was growing up, my family and doctors were obsessed with my health and always warned me not to overexert myself. Josh didn't pay any attention to what the doctors said. He saw me as a friend and a competitor, not some sick kid.

By the sixth grade, my mom thought I needed a change and I transferred to a public school closer to home. My biggest fear with this was that I would lose Josh's friendship, but Josh and I still hung out after school and on the weekends. We both found new friends, but no one who could take the place of the other.

Josh and I were reunited in high school. I went on to letter in tennis at Dunwoody High School, and was the only freshman to make the team in 1988. I'm proud to say that I was undefeated in doubles in eighteen matches in my four-year career. Josh, my adversary at the round robin, was my primary partner. We even knocked off Tucker High School, the defending state champions.

As we progressed through high school, Josh and I continued to be friends, but there were changes. We didn't have the same classes, nor did we go to lunch at the same time. Josh became friends with the cheerleaders, student council representatives and the popular crowd. Mostly, I hung with guys who didn't fit in. It was difficult to see the many friendships that Josh built when I had only a couple of buddies.

For the most part, my high school experiences were filled with confrontations with bullies, awkwardness around the opposite sex and pressures to be like everyone else. I didn't get invited to a lot of high school parties until my senior year. I did go to our senior prom, which was my first real date with a girl. I was a slow starter who never really fit in.

There were plenty of bullies who picked on me in high school, and even though I had become somewhat athletic, I was the ultimate poster boy for weak kids who could not defend themselves. First, there was Dexter. He used to drop his books on my head as his locker was above mine. He did it for three months until my mom got him suspended. Dexter never messed with me again. That's when Satchel took the bully role. He was an eighth grader who probably weighed 250 pounds. Satchel hazed me for about a year before I finally punched him in the stomach. I don't think I hurt him, but my punch combined with his hand grabbing my neck, brought over our gym coach. There were no more altercations after that.

Finally, there was David. He bullied me in the cafeteria by pushing my books onto the floor, dumping my lunch into the garbage and then laughing. It still stings when I remember how other kids laughed with him at my expense. And each time I got rid of a bully, another one came along. It was as if I had put an ad in the school paper—*Wanted: A big guy who doesn't take no for an answer. Must like to pick on someone smaller. Must be willing to resort to violence. See small skinny kid for further details.* Both my grades and my confidence slipped.

Mom knew something was wrong, but I wouldn't tell her what it was. It was my battle, and I was going to fight it myself. Josh tried to help. He and I went over our karate moves together. We'd both taken Tae Kwan Do at a local club, but Josh was much better than I was. I was frustrated and that frustration built until one time when David tried to grab my lunch. I shouted "No!" He pushed me.

"Give it to me," he demanded.

Then he saw the principal coming and pretended to stroll away. After that, he stopped bothering me.

As a scrawny kid who couldn't fight, I did what I had to do to survive. I took the teasing and I let my parents and teachers fight for me. While I may have been competitive, I lacked courage. Cystic fibrosis played a huge role in that and I became fearful . . . of everything.

Yet as college got closer, I grew excited. I wanted to change my image. I applied to four schools—Georgia Tech, Emory, The University of Georgia and the University of North Carolina. I applied to the first three because I wanted to be near home in case of emergencies and I applied to North Carolina because Dr. Boat was close. I knew my SATs would make it difficult for a good school to accept me. I was not a good test taker. My grades were solid but my SATs were middle of the pack. Thus, I did not get into Emory or North Carolina, but I was offered a spot in Emory's program at Oxford, a small Georgia town east of Atlanta. I could transfer to Emory in a couple of years if I did well, but I didn't want to go to a small school like Oxford. My father thought Emory was not the school for me, anyway. He knew my love for sports and thought I should go to a school where I could attend college football games on Saturdays. I did get into both Tech and the University of Georgia. Georgia Tech was more of an engineering school, and I knew that was not the direction I wanted to go. I'd visited Georgia many times and I loved the campus, especially on game day. There was no place like Athens, Georgia on a Saturday in the fall. I'd made my decision.

Both Mom and Dad were nervous about sending me off to school. I think every parent has mixed feelings about that, but my parents, obviously, had a lot more to worry about. And their worries were well-founded.

I started at the University of Georgia (UGA) in the fall of 1991. Like most freshmen, I was excited about the independence I'd finally have and the friends I expected to make, but I was also nervous. In addition to the usual jitters, I had a bunch of CF-related concerns: What if my therapy machine got strange looks from the people in my dorm? What if I got sick? What if I had a problem with my medicine? There were no cystic fibrosis specialists in Athens, at least not to my knowledge.

I'd hoped to sneak my therapy machine into the dorm, but it's hard to sneak in something that's three feet high and two feet wide with plastic hoses protruding from it. I could see people whispering to each other, and I guessed at what they were saying: "Hey, look, that kid must be really sick to need something like that." "What do you think that thing is? Why does he have to bring it to school?" and "Do you think he's contagious?"

While my mom made sure that every teacher I had from preschool on knew I had cystic fibrosis, I'd never told anyone—except Josh. I didn't want sympathy. And I didn't plan to tell anyone now. When someone inquired about the machine, I said it was my computer. It was a lame answer, but they didn't ask any more questions. I wondered if this experience were an omen, a hint of what my four years at UGA would be like . . . people giving me strange looks and laughing at me.

Before I left for college, my dad asked me what I wanted to study. I had no idea. Not a clue. He also asked if I thought about joining a fraternity. I admitted I didn't know much about them.

"It's like a club," my dad said, "but the members are called brothers. They're the guys who will be at your wedding and maybe even your son's bar mitzvah."

"I've got friends to hang out with."

"It's not the same," Dad said. "These guys are going to be your friends for life."

That expression stuck with me. The way he looked at me when he said "friends for life" made me realize his fraternity—he was a Phi Epsilon Pi at the University of South Carolina—had meant a lot to him, and still did. I figured I'd check it out.

I knew I already had a friend for life, but I wasn't sure if Josh would end up at Georgia. I thought with his grades he'd end up at a private school in the North, but fortunately he loved UGA, and he too landed in Athens. Best of all, we were going to be roommates.

Chapter 11
A Rush Decision

Josh and I attended fraternity rush and went from house to house meeting the brothers. We were put into different groups for a bus tour around campus. I was concerned because I wasn't the most social guy in the world and I didn't know a lot of people. It was a bit awkward. I envisioned the scene in Josh's bus with everyone gathered around patting him on the back as they laughed at his jokes.

As we walked into the fraternities, I saw trends develop. The sons of alumni were taken immediately to meet the brothers. Others, like me, were forced to have fake conversations with guys we knew did not want us to be part of their fraternity. Still, it was a great chance to brush up on my social skills.

Each of the brothers gave the same speech about their respective fraternities: "We have a nice house. We do well in academics. We are great in athletics." Blah, blah, blah.

The first house I visited that had any remote interest in me was Alpha Epsilon Pi, which was the "cool" Jewish fraternity. At least, that's what I heard from several of my peers. This time I was one of those taken to the back. The brothers there urged me to join, and quickly gave me a pen to sign my bid. It took me by surprise that after only five minutes they wanted me to be a brother for the next four years. I was ready to sign when I remembered there was another Jewish fraternity on campus. I asked the AE Pi brothers about it and one guy laughed.

"Yeah, there's Tau Epsilon Phi, but you don't want to join them. They're a bunch of losers," a guy named Michael said with a snicker.

I usually give in pretty easily to peer pressure, but that day I didn't. I felt I should weigh all my options before making such an important decision, so I told them I'd check out the other fraternity and if they were right, I'd be back. Michael didn't seem to like that answer.

"C'mon, man. Just sign," he said, sliding the bid card closer to me. "Don't be a loser, man."

If this place is so great, I thought, then why are they working so hard to convince me to join?

The next day I visited Tau Epsilon Phi. I got directions from a guy who said if I walked a half-mile down Baxter Street, I'd see the house.

"How will I know which one it is?" I asked.

He laughed. "You'll know it when you see it."

I walked a half-mile and didn't see any fraternity house. The directions I received were nowhere near fraternity row, so I began to wonder if the guy was playing a prank on a naïve freshman. I did pass a decrepit home that looked like a war relic waiting for the demolition crew. The columns on the porch were askew, and some bricks were missing from the façade. The windows were cracked. The roof looked as if it were made of rocks and loose wire. In the back, I could see a basketball goal two feet too short with a bent rim. I noticed a lot of people in the yard and wondered why they were gathered at a condemned house. Then I saw three letters on the front: T-E-P.

The interior was a perfect match for the exterior. As I entered the house, I heard a girl squeal, "Was that a rat?" The floor looked as if it hadn't been mopped since 1969, and some of the benches in the dining area were short a leg. The pool table was missing several balls, but didn't lack cigarette or beer stains. The closets were all locked, but I could hear something rattling in one of them. The only redeeming feature was the ice machine. It made the clearest, freshest cubes of ice I'd ever seen.

If I'd judged a book by its cover, I would have grabbed a cab from TEP, rushed over to AE PI and signed. I had a negative vibe from Michael, though, so I decided to give the TEP brothers a shot. After losing two plastic knives in the span of five minutes to a lunch of the rubberiest steak I'd ever eaten, I met all the brothers. I was surprised how nice they were. When I told them I was considering joining their rival, Alpha Epsilon Pi, I expected them to sneer and make crude remarks about them, but they didn't.

One of the brothers said, "TEP is great, but you have to choose which fraternity makes you happiest."

That took a lot of pressure off me. For the first time since I'd walked onto the University of Georgia campus, I felt comfortable. I spent several hours there, talking with them about standard guy stuff: women, sports and cars.

Maybe TEP could be a second home for me. Of course, I'd always prefer my parents' place because their bathroom had little things the fraternity bathroom was lacking, like toilet paper, towels and soap.

As I walked home, I thought about which fraternity I'd pledge. Would it be Alpha Epsilon Pi, the coolest Jewish fraternity on campus, or would it be Tau Epsilon Phi, which had an amazing ice machine? Josh and I talked it over that night and again the next morning. We both decided on TEP because the brothers were genuine, even if they weren't the coolest people in the world. Hey, I wasn't exactly the big man on campus either.

It was important to me to be part of a Jewish fraternity because I didn't have a lot of Jewish friends in elementary school. I went to a Presbyterian school from kindergarten to fifth grade. In public school there were more Jews, but still not a high percentage. I wanted to know more people who grew up with the same culture and traditions as I did.

We returned to the TEP house to tell our new brothers our decision. They grinned, slapped us on the back and shook our hands. We sat and chatted for several hours, and I knew I'd made a good decision.

We arrived the next week for our first pledge meeting. After waiting a while, a guy finally came up to us and screamed, "Sit down and shut up, you low-life pledges!"

"What the heck is going on?" I thought.

Pledging, we learned, was a humbling and occasionally humiliating experience. Whatever the brothers told us to do, we did. They didn't physically hurt us, but they did devise lots of schemes to embarrass and exasperate us. We had to call each other by our pledge names. Mine was "Cyrano." I wasn't too familiar with Cyrano de Bergerac, but I'd seen Roxanne and I knew the brothers were mocking my rather, uh . . . prominent . . . nose, which was one of my biggest insecurities. We had to memorize each brother's hometown, major and interests, and learn fraternity trivia and stats about famous football moments at the University of Georgia.

The brothers put other pressures on us, too. When our grades weren't up to snuff, the brothers explained that TEP was one of the top academic fraternities on campus and bad grades brought the fraternity down. Pledges who didn't bring dates to football games had to serve food and drinks. Some nights they even made us reenact plays from the Georgia game we just saw. We also did something called "Running the Shoot" where we had to find the best-looking girls who walked by our house and invite them to band parties at the fraternity house. The brothers usually picked the better-looking pledges to do this, so I rarely was chosen. Quite honestly, I was relieved because I was still uncomfortable with the opposite sex.

I always felt that between doing my therapy, pledging and trying to find my way around campus, I had very little time to study. My grades reflected this, as my GPA was below 2.0 my first two quarters at Georgia and I was placed on academic probation. One more quarter like that and I'd be out of school for good.

Sometimes I'd ask myself, "What's the point of pledging?" I didn't want to quit, though the brothers would have understood, I think. On our pledge sheets, we had to disclose any illnesses and an emergency contact, so they knew I had cystic fibrosis. They often asked if I was overburdened by the pledge demands and told me it was okay to miss a pledge meeting, if necessary.

I wasn't used to having people give me an out because I had CF. The only other time that happened was when my mom was writing notes to excuse me from gym class. I couldn't use cystic fibrosis as a crutch, though. I was going to be a brother in Tau Epsilon Phi by doing everything my fellow pledges did. I didn't want to be treated any differently. I also realized I was building friendships with my pledge brothers. I was finding, as my dad called them, "friends for life."

Chapter 12
Extreme Makeover—Andy Edition

Not long after I became a TEP pledge, I went with a bunch of pledge brothers to lunch at the cafeteria. Though I was among guys I thought were my friends, I was miserable. Everyone was ridiculing me.

At the time, I had a nondescript haircut that was perpetually out of control. My shirts were two sizes too small when oversized clothing was fashionable. I never bought new clothes—that was my mom's job. I still wore the blue jeans she'd picked out for me at Kmart. I wore a ratty pair of gray tennis shoes I'd had since my sophomore year of high school. I was no fashion plate. I knew this, but I really didn't think much about it until these guys began picking apart every aspect of my appearance.

I didn't defend myself because I was afraid that the only way I could compensate for my shortcomings was to do whatever my pledge brothers asked. Then they'd hang out with me. I always felt that because of CF, I had to go the extra mile to make friends. I knew it had to be tough on them because I was, after all, so different. So I listened to the guys tease me about how shy I was with girls and how I dressed like a geek. It wasn't the first time they'd said those things, and I was used to it. This day, though, one of my pledge brothers, Aaron Spitalnick, said something that cut me to the core: "Andy, man, the only reason people hang out with you is that you have a car and you drive them everywhere." I'd driven everyone to the cafeteria that afternoon, in fact. Secretly, I was afraid that what he said was true. Not only was I being hazed by the brothers, but I'd somehow found a way to be hazed by my fellow pledges, too. I was so upset that I called Aaron a jerk and stormed out of the cafeteria. Let them find their own way home.

I drove back to the dorm, fell on my bed and cried. Was Aaron right? Was I so desperate to be liked that I was willing to sacrifice my self-esteem to have these people as friends? Why did people make fun of me? And why didn't Josh stand up for me? He's known me forever and never cared how I dressed. Maybe he, like me, was afraid of the opinions of our peers. He probably just wanted to fit in, too, even if fitting in meant not coming to his best friend's rescue. This was not the first time that my anger overwhelmed me. Just a few weeks earlier, I was so frustrated that I tossed Josh's miniature trampoline right into his microwave and broke our only means of cooking.

Later that day, Josh and another pledge brother came by to see me, but I kept my face in the pillow. Then the phone rang. It was Aaron. I refused to talk to him, but he said something to Josh, and Josh put the phone next to my ear. "Dude," Aaron said, "I'm sorry, but it's the truth."

"You're a jerk!" I yelled and hung up.

Several hours later, there was a knock at the door. I didn't answer it, but the knocking didn't stop. I wiped the tears from my face and opened the door. It was Aaron.

"What?" I asked, ready to shut the door in his obnoxious face.

"Look, dude, I'm just trying to help you out," he said. "You obviously lack self-esteem. You can't say 'no' to anyone. You don't know how to dress. You don't know how to talk to girls. You don't…."

"Okay," I interrupted him. "I get the point. Why don't you help me then?"

Aaron considered that for a second and pounced on the idea. "Well, okay, but you have to be willing to make some drastic changes."

I was surprised that Aaron agreed, and wondered what changes he wanted to make. I had no social life, no girlfriend and no self-esteem. Basically, I had nothing to lose. "I'll do it," I said. "Let's get started."

That night, Aaron went through my closet item by item and removed everything I had that wasn't cool. He took every T-shirt I had, saying, "They make you look like a tool." (A "tool" is a synonym for a dweeb or geek.) He also ditched my caps, my white underwear, my white socks, my tennis shoes, every pair of shorts I owned, all my collared shirts and my sports memorabilia. "Never wear stuff with sports logos," he warned, "and never wear plain white socks." I didn't know where he got these rules or if they made any sense, but I nodded anyway. By the time he was done, I had one T-shirt, a few pairs of cotton boxers, a plain baseball cap, a pair of ripped-up khaki shorts and a pair of running shoes.

Aaron also told me that if I wanted a girlfriend, I'd need to get rid of my sports posters and bathing suit calendar. The calendar pictures intimidate girls, and they think sports posters are immature, he said. Whatever. I asked if I could keep Miss March. Aaron laughed and shook his head. I told him I was a big Braves fan and emphasized that they were in the midst of their infamous worst to first campaign, but he reminded me that if I wanted a girlfriend, I'd have to make some sacrifices.

He also suggested I change my attitude and style: Keep your head up and make eye contact with girls. "Don't be afraid to talk to a girl," he said. "If she doesn't like you, forget about her. Move on. Nobody is better than you."

I never forgot that. He told me to stop telling so many stupid jokes, because they made me sound like a moron. Honestly, though, I'll never be cured of that habit, and some of them are pretty funny.

Aaron also suggested I stand up for myself and say no every now and then. "The most important thing," he concluded, "is always to . . ."

"I know, I know," I said. "Always be myself."

He stared at me like I had three eyes. "Heck, no! What are you, an idiot?"

I think he was kidding.

The next day, I borrowed clothes from Aaron so I wouldn't have to go to class naked. That afternoon we went to the mall for my "makeover." At the mall I tried on more clothes than Claudia Schiffer at a fashion shoot. Some of the things he liked I never would have bought.

"Aaron, these jeans are too tight. I can't feel things I should be able to feel."

"That means they're perfect," he said with a nod. "We'll take them."

We bought three short-sleeved shirts with collars, two pair of khakis, a green wool cap, two long-sleeved collared shirts, two pair of jeans, some nice socks and a bottle of Obsession cologne. When my mom got the bill a month later, she asked if the credit card had been stolen.

I hadn't spent that much money in a mall in all my previous eighteen years combined. I told her the truth, but by the time she was done scolding me, I wished I had lied. It was the first time I'd bought clothes without my mother's help. It was also one of the first times that someone at school had done something nice for me and expected nothing in return.

Spending time at the mall made me think about the dream, the one where I was hiding under a clothes rack and Wendy asked if I needed help. Maybe she wanted to help me change my wardrobe, my image and my attitude. Could that be how she wanted to help me?

That night I made my debut at a TEP house party. I strolled in wearing hiking boots, a new pair of jeans, a green wool cap and a beige long-sleeve collared shirt over a T-shirt. The scent of Obsession floated through the air. I got looks—not the same kind of looks as when I wheeled my therapy machine into the dorm—of smiles and nods.

Someone laughed and asked if I was Aaron's protégé. I took it as a compliment because if I was going to take after someone, Aaron wasn't a bad choice. Aaron got a lot of razzing because of his cockiness. With Aaron, the cockiness was a front. Yes, he was confident, sometimes overly so, but he was a good person.

When Josh saw me, he said, "You're dressed like the ultimate fraternity guy. We're going to have to call you 'Fraternity Lipman.'" That eventually got shortened to "Flip," which my fraternity brothers call me to this day. It's a heck of a lot better than "Cyrano."

I had a great time at that party. I felt less self-conscious, so I mingled with everyone, even girls from the Jewish sororities. I felt better and got respect in return. Maybe it was my style (or lack of it) that made me feel different, not cystic fibrosis. I hoped things would be different from now on.

Aaron and I became close friends as a result of our shopping excursion. I liked him because he took a real interest in me and because he wasn't bothered by the fact that I had CF. When people learned I had CF and got that polite, concerned look on their faces, Aaron would interject, "Yeah, he can't breathe or anything. I think he's missing a lung. Does anyone see it? I hope he didn't lose it in the Jell-O again." When I'd be doubled over with a coughing attack, other people might nervously ask if I was okay. Aaron would ask if he should call the coroner.

That might sound cruel, but it was funny to me. I'd lived for so long with cystic fibrosis and dire reports about my health and life expectancy that it was a relief to hear someone joke about it. He wouldn't have joked about someone who was really sick or dying, and I was very much alive. When Aaron cracked jokes about CF, I'd think, "Hey, this isn't so bad. I can laugh at it. And I can beat it." It was through Aaron's humor that I finally got rid of the big elephant in the room.

Aaron helped transform my attitude about CF. I had always been secretive about it for fear that people would think I was odd or sick, but our friendship made me realize someone could like me for me. Aaron didn't care that I had CF any more than he cared that I was from Atlanta or a diehard Braves fan. It was one fact about me, but it didn't define me. At least, it didn't define me any more than I was willing to let it. That was an important lesson, but unfortunately, it was one I quickly forgot. Especially in the wake of bad news.

While I was learning to live my life at TEP, my best friend was losing his. Sadly, Howard died during my freshman year at college. To be honest, he should have died sooner, but I refused to let my mom take him to the vet to be put to sleep. By the time I left for college, he was blind and couldn't hear me when I called him. That broke my heart when I remembered how eager he'd been to be with me. At the end, he couldn't even lift his leg to pee. When he wanted to sit, he'd have to walk in a circle about ten times before he could lower himself to the ground. He'd wheeze from asthma. No longer was he the one running circles around the yard; I was now the more athletic of the two of us.

During my last year of high school, I made excuses about Howard's "accidents" in the house. I covered for him the way he covered for me. Imagine that, the sick kid taking care of the dog. Of course, he never saw me as the sick kid and I never saw him as a dog. He was just a friend who happened to have four legs and fur.

The night my mom called me to tell me Howard died, I was on my way to a fraternity party. I drank way too much that night, but it didn't numb my overwhelming sorrow over losing Howard, the dog who eagerly saved my life and never asked for a thing in return.

The next day, I decided I wouldn't wallow in grief when I thought about Howard. Instead, I'd remember his unconditional love and his eager brown eyes, and I would honor that memory by always celebrating his birthday. That decision numbed some of the sadness that enveloped me, but anyone who has ever lost a friend who happened to be a dog, knows that it never goes away entirely.

I mostly remember Howard when I'm on the softball field. I hustle between bases, remembering how he darted to my rescue and moved without an ounce of fear toward a bigger, dangerous opponent. I even wrote his name inside my glove. So far, no one has called me "Howard" or asked if that was my real name.

I still see Howard every now and then in my dreams. I can smell the funky scent of grass and fur and dog breath that is uniquely Howard, and I feel his warm breath on my face. It's a tremendous comfort to know that he is forever safe in my heart.

Some people ask me how a dog can mean so much. Those people obviously didn't own dogs and they never knew Howard. When you're battling a disease and you're tired of your parents being over-protective, you need a buddy who can just listen and let you vent. That was my Howard.

Chapter 13
Scared to be Different

By my sophomore year of college, everything began to come together. I felt comfortable on campus and knew lots of people. I moved from the dorm into the TEP fraternity house, as I was now a brother. After being on academic probation, I'd made a nice comeback and received Dean's List awards the next two quarters.

My room at TEP felt like home. Most of the rooms had lofts and mine, which was at the end of the hall, was no exception. My loft was elevated about five feet from the floor, so I had to duck to get into the room. To the left of the entrance was a two-foot wide closet without a door, and just past that was the loft. I had to duck under the loft to get to a dusty couch I'd bought at a used furniture store. My therapy machine was on the left in the back. The two windows were painted blue on the inside so they had to be open to see outside.

I hung a bikini calendar on the wall behind the couch. I knew the calendar was a no-no, according to Aaron, but there were some things I couldn't give up. There were all sorts of quotes written on and carved into the wood on the underside of my loft, which I could read looking up from the couch. Some might call these quotes graffiti, but for me they were messages sent from brothers who had been there in the early eighties. My favorite was, "Reach for the moon. Even if you miss, you'll still be among the stars."

Mom nearly had a stroke when she saw the place, but after five hours of cleaning, she felt a little better. Honestly, I didn't care. The room was comfortable and, more importantly, it was mine.

I was the only brother without a roommate. While I wanted a roommate, I found positives in having my own room. If I wanted to bring a girl back, I wouldn't have to worry about checking with my roommate. When I needed to do my therapy, I didn't have to worry if my roommate was asleep. Josh lived upstairs with a close friend from our pledge class. I was a little jealous, but I knew we couldn't live together forever.

My goal that year was to find a girlfriend. It was the only thing that seemed to be missing from my life. In the seventh grade, I liked a girl named Daphne, but we never went on an after-school "date," we never kissed, and we never even hung out, except in English class. She broke up with me because I was too embarrassed to tell my parents that I was going with her. I was always so shy and self-loathing that I never even kissed a girl until I got to college.

At college, the odds seemed to be in my favor. Some of the most beautiful women in the world were on the University of Georgia campus. I had a major crush on a girl named Helayne. Toward the end of my freshman year, I wrote poetry to her. The poetry was not romantic, but only because she was dating a fraternity brother of mine.

The summer after she broke up with him, she sprained her ankle during a softball game and I brought her a teddy bear. In addition to being beautiful—brown eyes, tanned skin and a cheerleader's athletic body—she was funny, sweet and easy to talk to. Basically, all she was missing was a halo. I'd fantasize about rescuing her from kidnappers or saving her life and winning her admiration, gratitude and eternal love. It sounds corny, but I wanted to be the hero. Yet I knew dating Helayne was unrealistic. I could see it in her eyes so I continued our friendship knowing it would never lead to anything.

It's always hard to deal with unrequited love, but it was especially hard for me because I didn't know if I'd ever find a girlfriend. Most of my fraternity brothers had girlfriends and I wanted the experience of a relationship, too. Not having one caused me to question my attractiveness to the opposite sex.

Still, I had a decent number of friends, and I was meeting more people. Things were going great, until one late night in the fraternity house. It was about two-thirty in the morning, and a bunch of brothers and some girls were watching a movie. I was finishing my therapy and my door was ajar, which was no big deal. My brothers were all used to the roaring sound of the machine, and they'd seen me wear the therapy vest and breathe the aerosols from the nebulizer. That's why I was able to relax with them. They knew I had cystic fibrosis and they accepted me for who I was.

As I was doing therapy, a girl I was interested in, and who I thought liked me, peeked in the room. A wave of what I took to be horror and disgust raced across her pretty face. I froze and then had a devastating thought, "She thinks I'm revolting. She thinks I look like an alien with all these freakish tubes attached to my body."

I had thought people accepted me and knew me as Andy, not as some freak. The change in wardrobe meant nothing. The person inside was still the same. I would always have cystic fibrosis. I was always going to have to use this machine, always take medications and always disgust women. I ripped off the vest and pulled the nebulizer from my mouth. "Get out!" I yelled. "Everyone get out!" I was crushed because I thought I had gained so much confidence. I had made so many new friends. My grades were improving, but seeing the girl's revulsion was as devastating as the time I read the encyclopedia article.

The elephant was back in the room. Hell, it had morphed into Godzilla.

Upon hearing my rant, several of my fraternity brothers rushed to my door and one asked, "What? What is it?"

I couldn't tell him.

When they left, I slammed the door shut and locked it. I snapped. I pounded on the door until my fist was sore. I hated this stupid machine. I hated myself. I hated this stupid disease. I hated my parents for giving it to me. I hated them all. I felt if one person thought I was different because of my CF, then everyone must think I was a freak. So many insecurities came to the forefront. Were people my friends because they liked me or because they pitied me? Was I ever going to meet a girl who thought of me as a man? Here I was in college dealing with my first opportunity to be on my own and being judged by my peers. Some people are prepared for that. I wasn't.

I threw the vest onto the floor and kicked the machine. Why do people have to be so ignorant? I wanted to die. God, just kill me already. I jammed my pillow on top of my head. I am a loser. I grabbed at my hair and pulled it out, strand by strand. I'll always be a loser and it's all because of cystic fibrosis. I don't want to face these people who think I'm a freak. Everyone pretends to like me, but they don't. They just feel sorry for me. God must hate me. He must really hate me to give me CF.

Chapter 14
CF Stands for "Crutch Found"

The next morning, I woke up with a sick feeling as I remembered what had happened the night before. Why even bother to get breakfast, I thought? I didn't want anyone to see me. I was sure all the girls thought I was grotesque. My friends probably thought so, too. That's why they're nice to me, I reasoned. They feel sorry for me because I have CF. I should have known that. Then I remembered the pledge football game we played toward the end of my freshman year.

It was the annual contest between our pledges and our archrivals, Alpha Epsilon Pi, the other Jewish fraternity. The rivalry between AEPI and TEP was heated, to say the least. While we were both Jewish fraternities, we'd been in many verbal confrontations, several fist fights, and had destroyed each other's property. Competing for the same kids every year to keep the money coming in was probably a big reason for the hatred. The football game was my chance to show my fraternity brothers and fellow pledges what I could do athletically, and it was a chance to impress the girls who'd be watching. I was eager to play, but a little puzzled because, during the weeks we were practicing, the coaches kept asking, "Do you need to take a break?" and "Are you sure you can do these exercises?" Of course I was sure.

I came to practice every day and memorized the plays. I worked on my defense. I worked on my offense. Each night before I fell asleep, I pictured myself catching the winning touchdown. My teammates would cheer and carry me off the field. The girls would all want me, and the guys would all want to be my friend.

The day of the game, the coaches told me I wouldn't be starting. That's okay, I thought. It's not who starts that matters—it's who finishes. But as the game progressed, my excitement began to wane. I wanted to play! By the fourth quarter, our team was down by two touchdowns. I might not be the hero, but at least I'd get to play, I thought. I put myself in the coaches' line of vision, figuring they couldn't possibly miss me, but they wouldn't look at me. The final seconds ran down and our team lost.

I wasn't one of the best players, but I was good enough to play. That I knew for sure. "Why didn't you put me in?" I asked a coach after the game.

"We didn't want you to get hurt. The fraternity can't risk a lawsuit," he said. That stung. I was devastated that I had been treated differently because I had CF. I was sick of standing on the sidelines. I wanted to participate with everyone else. I never begged off anything because of CF, or expected anyone to give me a break. So why did people insist on doing it?

Early one evening, a few days after I'd slammed the door on my fraternity brothers and alienated myself in my room, Josh knocked on my door.

"Let's go out," he hollered.

"Nah," I said. "I don't feel well. I'm tired." Josh and I were no longer inseparable buddies, but he still made an effort from time to time. The problem was that I had quit on everyone. I didn't want to see his face—or anyone else's.

"C'mon, man. We'll be back in a few hours and then you can go to bed."

"No, thanks. I don't feel well."

I faked a coughing spasm.

"All right, man. Feel better. Talk to you later."

I knew CF was good for something—making people feel sorry for me. I fell asleep, only to be awakened a few hours later by another knock.

"Dude, you home?" my fraternity brother Greg Green asked. "Let's go, man. The party's starting."

I didn't answer.

"C'mon man, let's go. Let's meet some chicks."

Just what I needed . . . bring me along so the girls can giggle about the hideous guy who connects himself to a life support machine. Obviously, if one girl knew, they all knew. They were probably discussing me now, trying to figure out how long I'd live. No wonder no one wanted to go out with me. I heard Greg knock again and then listened as his footsteps grew softer. Finally I heard the main door open then slam shut. Aaron was next as he tried to get me out of my funk by nearly beating the door down, but I refused to come out. Other brothers knocked, too, but soon the knocking stopped. No one bothered to check on me anymore. It was pointless. I was not budging.

I realized I hadn't eaten in nearly twenty-four hours, but I didn't want to go to the kitchen because everyone would ask where I'd been and why I was hiding. The last thing I wanted to do was run into the girl whose face contorted in disgust when she saw me using my therapy machine. I wasn't going to use it that night, I decided. I didn't want anyone to hear it running and the sound isn't easy to ignore. As there was a band party in the house, I knew there could be a couple hundred people.

My fear of people hearing my therapy machine reminded me of my freshman year. When I used the machine in the dorm, my neighbors would pound on the wall because it was so loud. I didn't want to tell them the machine was keeping me alive because I had a life-threatening genetic illness. I didn't want their pity. I did my part to look normal. I lied. I hid the machine in my closet under my dirty laundry. Still people knew, and still they stared.

By three-thirty in the morning, the band finally called it quits, the voices in the hall quieted and the only sound I could hear was the steady chirp of crickets. I went to the bathroom for the first time since the day before. I was hungry, but I decided to wait until morning to eat. No one would be sober enough to be up before noon.

At ten o'clock Sunday morning, I tiptoed from the house and headed to a nearby Shoney's restaurant, a place known for its breakfast food and buffet, but I was focused on my favorite dessert. I bought a twelve-inch strawberry pie and wolfed it down. I ate nothing else and skipped my therapy again. I couldn't remember ever skipping therapy. Doing it every day was such an ingrained part of my routine, like taking a shower or brushing my teeth. Other than taking pills, it was the only part of my daily life that reminded me I had CF. Skipping therapy made me feel, temporarily, like everyone else, and I rationalized that I got an extra thirty or forty minutes of my life back.

After two days without therapy, I began having trouble breathing. Every time I inhaled, I heard a rattle in my chest. I developed a cough that became deep and hacking, the way a hardcore smoker's cough sounds. I realized I had skipped my medication all weekend, too, and hadn't taken any vitamins or antibiotics. Because I didn't eat, I didn't take my Pancrease, a medication that helps my pancreas digest fatty foods. Yet, I decided to wait, and take my medication and do my therapy on Monday.

When I woke up on Monday, I couldn't stop coughing. My chest was throbbing and my throat was hoarse. I was coughing so badly I couldn't walk to class. I made my way outside, but I had to stop and bend over because the coughing spasms made it impossible to stand. I decided to skip my classes. I could afford to miss a day and rest, and I knew I could tell the instructor I had CF. She'd surely feel sorry for me, combating a life-threatening illness. It was as if I were back in grammar school, using cystic fibrosis as a crutch so I could skip gym class.

That night I did my therapy, thinking I'd feel better. I didn't. In fact, I'd never felt worse.

The next day I skipped classes again. I was still congested and my sides ached from coughing, but thought I could play basketball. As soon as I started, though, I realized how wrong I was. I began coughing up huge chunks of phlegm. It was a light green color, which scared me because my doctors had warned me if it's anything but clear, it means I have an infection.

My teammates, the guys who were supposed to be my friends, asked me if I was going through puberty because my voice was so hoarse. I couldn't stand it anymore! I was sick-and-tired of people making fun, of girls avoiding me, of the rude stares and the even ruder jokes. I yelled two words I never thought I'd say: "I quit!"

I had never felt like quitting before. Quitting was like doing drugs or shoplifting—things I'd never even consider. Even when I tried out for the fraternity softball team as a freshman and the captain told me I probably wouldn't displace any of the returning seniors for a spot on the team, I didn't quit. I didn't make the team, but I did the best I could. Quitting was new to me. Depressed, I rationalized this situation was not my fault. My doctors had told me that as cystic fibrosis patients got older, their bodies deteriorated. This was normal.

As if to prove my doctors right, my coughing was getting worse, my stamina was decreasing, and my phlegm was turning bright green. I knew I should see a doctor, but felt I shouldn't bother to pay good money just to hear the inevitable—that my days were numbered.

Chapter 15
Doctor Doom

My life was falling apart. I stopped socializing, barely went to class, and used my therapy machine irregularly. I took my meds on days I felt like it, which wasn't often. Mostly, I sat in my room, listened to music and slept.

Six weeks after I'd isolated myself from society, Mom and I drove to Chapel Hill for my biannual appointment with Dr. Boat. When I took the pulmonary function test—a key procedure in determining my health, where I blow into a tube three to eight times to gauge my lung function—I expected my breathing capacity would be as impressive as it had been since Dr. Boat became my doctor. Feeling so sick, I should have expected poor results, but I'd rarely seen my pulmonary function scores drop since I began seeing Dr. Boat. Usually the test administrator would examine my results and say, "Wow! You have CF? No way." This time, though, she didn't say anything as she made a notation on my chart. I asked for another chance, but I did even worse. The third time was my worst score, and afterward, I felt light-headed to the point I feared I'd pass out.

A nurse examined me and asked the same questions she always did. I knew if I admitted anything that had been going on they'd haul my butt into the hospital, where in my current apathetic state, I'd probably die. If I gave the usual answers to the questions, maybe they'd just let me go home, so I lied.

"Are you spitting up phlegm?"

"Uh, not really."

"When you do, what color is it?"

"Usually clear."

"Nothing green or yellow?"

"Nope."

"Are you coughing a lot?"

"No, just the usual amount."

She looked at me suspiciously.

"Do you feel pain in your chest when you cough?"

God, yes, I thought to myself.

"No."

I wished my dad had been there. Usually he came with us, but he'd been called away on a business trip. He would know what to do if he were here.

The instant Dr. Boat entered the room, I knew something was seriously wrong. Unlike the other times I'd seen him, he seemed reluctant to speak with us. "Well," he finally said, "I looked at Andy's X-rays, and we need to make some changes immediately, before the bacteria in his lungs spreads."

He looked at me and said, "Your health isn't as good as it was the last time we met."

No kidding.

"I'm not sure why."

I wasn't going to volunteer any information. I'd become an expert at keeping secrets about myself and I was not going to change my approach now.

"The X-rays show a definite inflammation in Andy's lungs," he said, turning to my mom. "We'll have to do a sputum culture to see if it's pseudomonas."

My mother's terrified eyes darted to Dr. Boat's face. "Pseudomonas? Do you think it's that?"

"All I'm saying is it's a possibility," he said calmly.

I'd heard the word "pseudomonas" mentioned before, but I knew very little about its severity. Judging from my mom's reaction, it was quite serious.

Dr. Boat listened to my chest. "There's definitely some obstruction there." He went to his table and scanned my chart. "Your pulmonary function scores are down considerably. We'll have to change some of your medicines. Let's see . . . are you getting a lot of exercise?"

What was I going to say? That I lie in my bed for forty-eight hours at a time, sometimes without eating a thing? Oh, and over the last six weeks I did my therapy maybe three times a week and I no longer take most of my medications. Of course I couldn't tell him that. He'd freak out. My mom would freak out. She'd yank me out of college.

"Oh, yeah," I said. "I play basketball. Tennis. Softball. And football. Every sport. Never felt in better shape."

I would've said I played Australian Rules football if it would rip that suspicious look off Dr. Boat's face. I knew he didn't believe me. In my brain, a chorus shrieked, "I'm going to die. I'm going to die. I'm going to die." Could my mom hear it? I looked at her, hoping she'd reassure me, but she didn't say anything. Tears filled my eyes. I discretely wiped them away.

"I think he's scared, Dr. Boat. Can you tell him he can get better?"

Gee, thanks, Mom. That's what you call support?

Dr. Boat's face softened a little. "Andy, we're going to do everything we can to get to the bottom of this and get you back on track," he said. "If you take care of yourself, you should be fine."

How reassuring. Why not measure me now for the casket? What's with the "should be fine?" It sounded like he knew something I didn't, and that can only be something bad. I'm going to die. I am truly a failure. Ever since I was little, doctors used words that made the most positive sentence bleak.

"Andy should be fine . . . for now."

"Andy, you shouldn't have anything to worry about . . . at this point."

In my head, I knew they meant, "Things are fine now, but some day they'll be much worse."

Dr. Boat prescribed some strong antibiotics and an inhaler. Just what I needed, something else to make me look like a freak. He said he wanted to see me again soon, but I knew that the next time he'd see me it would most likely be for the autopsy. The pessimism in the room crushed my chest. No wonder I had difficulty breathing.

We got in the car for the long ride home, and my mom said, "We'll get through this." But her eyes, framed in the rear-view mirror, were sad. "Just take better care of yourself. Do your therapy twice a day. Take the new prescriptions. Things will get better. You'll see."

That was just my mom being a mom. I knew she was frightened, and I thought she was putting on a front so I wouldn't be more afraid than I already was. I remembered the encyclopedia article that said I'd be dead by twenty-five and the CF movies with the sad endings. That was the reality for most people like me. Thinking I would live a long, normal life—well, that was the fantasy. I just didn't want to accept it . . . until now. "Andy, it's OK," my mom said again. No it isn't, I thought. I'm going to die. I hate you. I hate everyone. Leave me alone.

Emily was clamoring for Chicken McNuggets, so Mom pulled into a McDonald's.

"I'm staying in the car," I said.

"Don't be selfish. Your sister needs to eat."

Then I thought, me, selfish? You must be kidding. I'm the one who's sacrificing my life to this stupid disease.

Emily, oblivious to what was happening, opened the car door and was skipping toward the restaurant, waving to us to hurry up. Emily was an energetic, happy seven-year-old, who knew very little about cystic fibrosis.

I didn't move. My mother began to cry. "Please, Andy. This isn't easy for me, either."

I started crying too. The sight of my mom in tears always does that to me. But I refused to feel sorry for her just because mascara was smeared on her face. She wasn't the one who was suffering.

"I don't care if I die," I sobbed. "You don't care either. Dad doesn't care—he's not even here."

"I do care, and so does Dad," said Mom. Her eyes met mine with a hard glance. "Stop feeling sorry for yourself. It will do you no good. Let's eat."

"I don't want to eat. I don't need to eat. I'll die faster if I don't eat."

My mother sighed in exasperation. "Andy, please. I can't take this anymore. You're not being fair to me."

"Fair to you?" I cried. "You think this is fair to me? You gave me this stupid disease! How do you think I feel? Just leave me alone! Let me die in peace!"

My mother let out a wrenching cry that cut into my heart. To this day, I vividly remember the great, heaving sobs that made her shoulders shake and her head bow in grief. I'd never seen her weep like that before. Tears dripped onto her blouse, leaving little opaque circles. I knew what I said hurt her more than anything I'd ever uttered. No doubt she did blame herself for the fact that her son had CF. No doubt she had spent many nights fearing exactly what I feared and putting on a brave face so I wouldn't be afraid. She'd lost Wendy, and she was terrified that I was next.

I wanted so much to tell her I was sorry and I wanted her to hold me and rock me like she did when I was little. I wanted to beg her to make everything better, like she always used to do with a Band-Aid and a kiss. But I couldn't do it. I still clung to the resonating anger I felt in Dr. Boat's office, and I was too preoccupied with my own sad state of affairs to give much thought to how I'd wronged anyone else.

That afternoon, my mother and I did not breathe a word as my sister played on the McDonald's playground. After lunch, we drove back to Georgia in silence. Since that day, my mother has never accompanied me to Dr. Boat's office. From that day on, it was my father's job.

I thought about my body's steady deterioration. I could be dead before I graduated from college. I didn't want to go back to school. My "friends" already thought I was a loser. I hadn't been to class in weeks. I knew I was failing calculus. I hated my life and I hated myself. I couldn't think of a thing to look forward to.

When Mom dropped me off at the fraternity house she preached how important it was that I follow Dr. Boat's orders to the tee. She was reluctant to let me go back to school, but I think she knew it would only be worse at home. As she and Emily drove off, I watched her car vanish beyond the hill. One question suddenly popped into my head: Would that be the last time I saw my mother?

Chapter 16
A Nightmarish Return

When I got back to school, I did what I always did—went straight to bed. I was obsessed by thoughts of death and dying; I really couldn't think about anything else. When I managed to sleep, it was never for long. Coughing spasms woke me repeatedly during the night. I sat in the dark hacking up huge chunks of phlegm. I stopped answering the phone and the door. This no longer seemed strange to me. It really didn't matter though because no one knocked on my door anymore and other than my mom and Aunt Susie, no one called. I wanted to be left alone to die. I wanted people to feel guilty for the way they treated me.

I especially wanted Josh to feel that way. Josh was the one person I felt I could always count on and confide in, but lately I felt our friendship slipping away. Instead of spending time with me, he was busy with his new girlfriend. To make matters worse, my fraternity brothers had been bragging that since Josh began working out, he was irresistible to women. The guy now had a six-pack that rivaled any bodybuilder's.

During this time, I remember watching a video with a girl who I thought really liked me. I'm not sure how that happened, as I rarely ventured from my room unless I had to go to class, and often not even then. This girl knew I had CF but didn't seem to care. That was a great sign as far as I was concerned. I still had hopes I could find a girlfriend. A girlfriend, I thought, would go a long way in making life better. But as we watched, she asked if I knew when Josh would be home and if he were seeing anyone. Then she asked if I thought he'd go out with her. I was crushed. She obviously wasn't hanging out with me because she was interested in me. I remembered when Josh and I were so alike that people used to mix us up. Now he had become a stud and I'd become a dud.

I stopped going to parties. A couple times I thought about showing up, but when I gripped the doorknob, I'd hear voices in the hall and lose my nerve. I'd creep back to my couch and put a pillow over my head. I was afraid people would see me and remember what a freak I was. The longer I spent in my room, the harder it became to leave. I felt more and more isolated and didn't know how to break out. Honestly, I wasn't sure I wanted to.

In October of that year, my beloved Braves were playing in Game 7 of the National League Championship Series against the Pittsburgh Pirates. It was the most exciting game in the team's history. They trailed 2-1 in the ninth with the tying run at third base, and the winning run at second base. There were two outs. When Francisco Cabrera, a little known player, knocked a game winning single to send the Braves to their second straight World Series, I could hear the bedlam coming from the neighboring rooms as my fraternity brothers celebrated together. Each of them would remember where he was when Cabrera knocked in Bream to win the pennant. The only recollection I would have would be shutting off the television, sitting all alone in the dark and choking as thick gobs of green phlegm stuck to the back of my throat.

At night I listened to Jimmy Buffet's "Feeding Frenzy," hoping his laid-back vocals would inspire me. I rented inspiring sports videos like *The Karate Kid* and *Rocky*, with the same hope. They didn't work, either. All they did was remind me of how far I'd sunk after being such an accomplished athlete. At the time, I didn't think I was destined to be someone who was counted out, and then came back to win the fight. I was on the ropes and no one, especially not me, was going to come to my rescue. The days dragged on. I felt less than alive.

I knew something was desperately wrong. I needed to talk to someone, but had no reliable confidant. I considered going to a psychiatrist, but the only way I had of paying for sessions was with my parents' credit card. As soon as they saw the bill, they would know I was in a crisis. As much as I needed help, I didn't want to admit any weakness to them. I felt it would only confirm that I should never have gone away to school because I obviously couldn't manage to care for myself.

I spiraled into an even deeper depression, and I soon lost all will to fight it. I continued skipping therapy. The drugs Dr. Boat prescribed sat unopened on my dresser. I talked to almost no one. When my mom called, I'd quickly wrap up conversations by telling her I was getting ready to go out with friends. That way she wouldn't have a chance to sense that something was wrong. I knew I couldn't have talked to her for long without sobbing for help. On weekends I hid in my room, telling my fraternity brothers I was going home. I never went to the grocery store or to the dining room. I basically starved myself. I even began parking my car blocks from the fraternity house so no one would know I was home.

Since I'd alienated my old group of friends, I fell into a different crowd. I spent time with guys who did poorly in school and had problems themselves. One of my brothers hated the fraternity because everyone accused him of stealing. I knew the feeling of being treated like an outsider, I said with a nod.

Another fraternity brother used to go with me to the convenience store. He was big, about six-foot-three and 250 pounds, and displayed his internal rage when he told how life had treated him so unfairly. He said his parents had all but abandoned him and he was in love with a married woman. He confided that he'd like to climb to the top seats of the football stadium and hurl himself over the side. We talked about suicide on several occasions. The way he described it, I could imagine myself doing it. I truly thought I could die that way. I don't know if he was serious about killing himself, but I became obsessed with the idea.

I envisioned buying a gun and blowing my brains out, or buying yards of strong rope, tying a noose and hanging myself. The next morning, Josh would come in and find my lifeless body hanging from the ceiling in the bathroom. He'd be overcome with grief and remorse, thinking about all the times he hadn't been there for me. I wanted him to hate himself as much as I hated myself. I thought about death so much that I was no longer afraid of it. At that point in my life, death would have come as a relief.

My dreams were grim, with the exception of one. I continually dreamt that Wendy found me in the mall and asked if I needed help. "No," I told her. I didn't need her help. When I said that, she'd vanish. But she was persistent. She'd come back night after night, politely asking if I needed help. My answer was not honest, but it never changed. If only I'd known then who she was.

I slept fitfully. Night after night I'd wake in a cold sweat, which would mix with my tears of pain and the globs of mucous my body produced. I didn't sleep in my loft bed anymore. I slept on the sofa because I knew I would have to stumble to the shower to clean myself off. As I fumbled with the faucets and rinsed the filth from my increasingly emaciated body, I plotted as best I could. How could I get a gun? When and where would I kill myself? Who would really care if I were dead?

One evening when I wandered into the kitchen, one of the more popular brothers eyed me and said, "Hey, Andy, have you ever had sex? Are you gay?"

"No," I said.

A friend with him snorted and said condescendingly, as though he were talking to a kindergartener, "It's okay if you are."

I felt trapped. If I left, I'd look like I was running away because they were going to uncover some secret about me, and if I stayed, I'd have to endure more ridicule at a time when I was far too vulnerable to fight it. I froze.

"We'll get a prostitute for your birthday," one said with a laugh, and the others joined in.

"I don't want a prostitute," I said. I was quickly losing control of my emotions.

"Then you must be gay," he concluded.

"Screw all of you!" I yelled. Though I didn't want to cry in front of them, I couldn't help it. The tears fell anyway. I ran out of the kitchen and slammed the door. I briefly thought about the idea of sex with a prostitute. Who would want to have sex with someone with cystic fibrosis, even if she got paid for it? Who would want to be with me? No girl on the University of Georgia campus. That much I knew for sure.

I couldn't imagine things getting much worse, but indeed they did.

Chapter 17
The Final Straw

The only reason I didn't commit suicide was that I was afraid of the pain. I wish I could say that I didn't kill myself because I worried about how it would affect my little sister or how my parents would be destroyed, but that wasn't why I didn't do it. I was just afraid of the pain I would feel from the blast of a bullet through my head or the pain my neck would endure when it snapped from a noose. Honestly, in the back of my mind, I hoped something good would happen that would change my situation. I was doing nothing to change things, but I felt I was owed a break from God. I struggled day-to-day, waiting for my break. Meanwhile things continued to get worse.

One afternoon, I couldn't find my accounting textbook. I thought maybe I'd misplaced it since I'd been skipping classes and hadn't used it for several weeks. I checked my backpack, the backseat of my car, my desk and under the bed. I didn't know where else it could be. I asked my two new loser friends, my only friends now, if they'd seen it. Both said no, so I went to the bookstore to buy another copy. Then I remembered a brief conversation I had with my two pals earlier that day and it stopped me cold. They told me they sold their textbooks right after final exams. I thought it was strange that moments after final exams the two of them didn't go celebrate. Instead, they went straight to the bookstore.

I asked a girl who worked at the bookstore if I could look at the accounting books they'd bought back that day. Sure enough, there was an accounting book from my class, and it had my notes in it. I asked who sold it to them, and they showed me the signature on the receipt. Sure enough, it belonged to the brother everyone had accused of stealing. Not only was he a thief, he was also a liar. I felt both betrayed and angry. I had trusted him and stood up for him when others accused him of stealing, and this was how he repaid me.

When I got back to the fraternity house, I confronted him, telling him I'd seen his signature on the receipt at the bookstore. Despite that evidence, he denied selling my book. He said he'd found the book in his room and assumed it was his. I knew that book had never left my room. He also failed to reimburse me for the cost of buying the book back.

I tried to have him removed from the fraternity, but I couldn't get enough votes. It wasn't even close. In other words, despite hard evidence the guy was a thief and a liar, my fraternity brothers sided with him rather than with me. That really hurt. Despite what the brothers said about being friends forever, each made it clear that I was being tolerated, nothing more. It didn't matter that I was the person who had clearly been wronged. To make matters worse, I had to see this thief every day, and though we didn't hang out anymore, he acted like nothing had happened. For some reason, I felt as if I had done something wrong in demanding he be removed from TEP. Somehow, I'd managed to become an outcast from a group of outcasts.

During my second and third years of college I had completely lost sight of who I was and what mattered to me. I really had no idea what purpose I had, if any. I wasn't enjoying college. I was barely surviving it. I even found things coming out of my mouth that I never thought I'd say, and before this despair would have been unthinkable to say. That depressed me even more.

I angered people left and right. One friend, Bert Rosenthal, told me how difficult it was for him to handle work and school. Bert is one of the hardest working people I know and definitely an over-achiever. If he was having trouble, what hope did I have? Bert told me I had no idea how tough it was because I wasn't working.

The old me would have brushed the comment aside. Instead, I bitterly replied, "Well, at least you'll be alive in ten years." There was absolutely nothing he could say in response, and I was glad. I deserved his pity. After all, I was dying. I'd gladly work twenty-four hours a day for the rest of my life in exchange for a life free of the death sentence of cystic fibrosis.

Another time, I was watching my fraternity brothers play basketball. I spotted a pledge brother, who everyone knew was having a tough time in classes. He was also having a tough time on the court. Instead of passing the ball to his teammates, he kept shooting it himself, which is not good strategy or team etiquette. I was in a foul mood, so I yelled, "Hey, you know the rules. No pass, no play"—which is what they tell student athletes whose grades are suffering. He stopped cold on the court and his face flushed with shame.

The other players looked at me and shook their heads. "You know he's not doing well this quarter," one said. "How could you say that?" someone else added.

My grades were nothing to impress, either. I'd missed weeks of class and had lost all interest in studying. One day, I had to get a ride to see my calculus professor because I was too weak to walk, though it wasn't far. I didn't drive my car because there was no place to park, so I begged rides from people who could drop me off. At the time, I hated being around or talking to people, but the thought of struggling to get to class was an even bigger concern. I was nervous about seeing my professor. I'd been gone so long she probably wouldn't even recognize me. I told the instructor how sick I'd been—this was obvious from looking at me—and how weak I was. I cried and embellished my story to make myself even more pitiful.

She seemed sympathetic and told me that if I did well on the final, she'd take my illness into account. What a relief. She wouldn't be able to live with herself if she failed someone who was dying. I was sure she'd give me a "C" out of pity. One less thing to worry about.

When I got my grades, my jaw dropped. I had two "C's" and an "F" in calculus. My "C" grades were in composition classes. The only reason I passed those was because of my gift for writing. I had never failed a class. Ever. I had no idea what I was going to tell my parents.

My father was angry, so I wisely never told him how many classes I'd skipped, how little I'd studied and how little I cared about anything. I explained that I'd always had a hard time with math, and I was sick a lot. He looked disappointed, but his mind was elsewhere. He was preoccupied with moving his own father into an assisted living center. All he said was to try harder next quarter.

I didn't try harder, though. The next quarter was just like the previous one. I skipped classes. I didn't have the stamina to drag myself to class, primarily because I was still skipping therapy and rarely taking my meds. On weekends I'd stay in my room with the lights off while fraternity parties downstairs rocked the house.

That quarter, one fraternity brother told me he knew what I could do to feel better. "You need to try pot," he said. This was something I never would have even thought of doing when I felt confident about my health, my athletic ability and my friends, but things were different now. I reasoned I had nothing to lose because I was going to die anyway. He said he'd just got a new stash and would be glad to share it with me the next night.

Though I knew nothing would change my mind, I called Aunt Susie to ask if marijuana could hurt me. My aunt and I had always had a special relationship. She even moved to Atlanta when I was small to help take care of me. She learned how to do my therapy and was a great confidant when I needed someone to talk to other than my parents. I knew how cool my aunt was so I figured the mention of marijuana would not evoke the kind of crazy reaction that I'd get from my mother. In this, however, I was wrong.

"Andy," she said, "don't be stupid. It could kill you. Promise me you won't do it."

I was taken aback by my aunt's reaction. I thought she was supposed to be cool about things like this. "Okay, I promise," I said. I knew I was lying to someone who loved me, but I didn't care.

Chapter 18
Knocked Down . . . But not Out

The next day, Monday, I woke at noon. This week would be like every other; there wasn't much to look forward to. I'd be skipping classes again. I'd spent the weekend hidden in my room crying and feeling sorry for myself, nourished only by a Shoney's strawberry pie. My cough had grown increasingly worse. The hacking was so loud at this point that I knew I was not fooling anyone about being out of town. I pulled myself out of bed, showered, dressed and made my way outside into the balmy fall afternoon. The sun was so bright I had to shade my eyes. I knew most of my housemates were at class, so I wouldn't have to deal with snide comments as I left my room for the first time in days. Little did I know that this was the day that would change my life.

As soon as I pushed open the outside door, I saw the guy who offered to share his pot with me. He was sitting in his car at the curb and waved to me to come over.

"Hey," he said, "I've got something to show you." He fumbled in the backseat and pulled out a baggie of marijuana. I tried to look blasé, as though I'd seen lots of pot before, but the truth was I'd never seen any illegal drugs up close.

"You excited about tonight?" he asked.

"Yeah, I guess."

"Good. It'll be cool. See you later."

I wandered over to the couch by our basketball court. I should have been in economics class, but I didn't want to go. I'd been to that class just once in the past three weeks, and I was afraid the instructor would notice my absence—or in this case, my presence. Instead, I sat soaking up the sun. I had nowhere to go and didn't care.

Before long, a group of brothers came out of the house with a basketball and began shooting baskets. It was a perfect day for a game, nearly 90 degrees and sunny, but not too humid. I envied their stamina and grace and remembered sadly how it felt to aim a jump shot and have perfect confidence that the ball would cleanly swish through the net.

"Ouch! I'm out!" someone yelled, interrupting my reminiscence as he limped off the court.

"Hey Andy," one of my pledge brothers said, "play." It was part request, part command.

No way, I thought. Do you guys want to lose? Yet I thought I might have a little game left in me, and what did it matter? "Okay," I said.

Almost instantly, I was exhausted. I coughed and wheezed and couldn't catch my breath. I was spitting up chunks of green phlegm. My shirt was soaked in sweat. The game seemed to last for hours. The sun, which had felt warm on the sofa, beat down on me. Finally our team got the ball. It was mine. I shot it. It was an air ball, a shot that went nowhere. I used to have what some of my fraternity brothers admiringly called "The Shot" because it was so accurate. I used to be able to shoot that shot floating out of bounds from twenty-five feet away. Now I couldn't make an eight-foot jump shot from the middle of the lane. "The Shot" was gone.

Toward the end of the game, I was taking breaks at every possession change and heaving up enough mucus for an entire sick ward. I was minutes from quitting when one of the fraternity's best players crouched for a jump shot. I tried to block him and the next thing I felt was a blow that sent me to the ground like a pin in a bowling alley. At first I didn't know what hit me, then I realized I'd been plowed over by a two-hundred-pound player named Brett, who was built like a wall. Between coughing spasms, I looked up from the ground to see him grinning maliciously.

His beefy hands encircled my skinny bicep and he lifted me off the ground. I had no power to resist him or to help myself up. I was like a marionette without strings, a limp version of myself.

"Entering any weightlifting contests soon?" Brett said with a sarcastic laugh. Everyone laughed with him. They were laughing at me, as usual. His jab took another cut into what little ego I had left. I was hurt yet again, and I realized I was angry, too. What right does he have to mock me like that? I thought.

Then suddenly, I realized Brett had every right. I was a loser who deserved to be scorned. I wasn't a loser because of CF, though. I was a loser because cystic fibrosis was my excuse for everything that sucked in my life, from my lack of friends and a girlfriend to my bad grades and even worse attitude. By telling myself I was a failure because I had CF, I made myself into one. No one used to care that I had CF. I was the one who let it define me to such a point that other people couldn't ignore it. Why hadn't I realized that before? I finished that basketball game. It hurt terribly. I gasped for breath with every shot, and my throat and chest felt raw and burned from incessant coughing. Still, I felt that standing on that court when the game ended was critical to a potential comeback. My team lost and I was the reason. After the game everyone headed inside to shower and eat dinner . . . everyone except me. I stayed on the deserted court, stared at the sky and searched for answers.

I remembered other games I'd played and how my fraternity brothers vied to have me on their team. I remembered when they didn't want to guard me because I was such an accurate shooter. Now they didn't want to guard me because there was no challenge in it. I was hardly an athlete and even less of a person. I was a sick kid with cystic fibrosis.

As I stared into space, questions swirled in my head: What had happened to me in the last year? How had I faded from the cool and athletic "Flip" to someone so self-hating and timid, so pitiful and despairing? I'd always had a steady stream of friends calling to invite me out or stopping by to talk. I'd chased them all away and retreated into myself. Was I any happier? No. Had I made peace with CF? Not really. So what was I doing? Where was I going?

I turned these thoughts over for so long that the afternoon faded to evening and the lights in the fraternity house and the houses across the street began to pop on. Finally, I pulled myself up from the sofa and slowly walked inside.

In my room, all the rage I'd been feeling for months welled up inside me. "What the hell have I done to myself?" I screamed. I was so enraged that I ripped off my shirt. "I hate myself! I hate myself! I hate myself!"

Then I said something I hadn't said or thought in all those months. I don't know where it came from, maybe it had been lurking in my subconscious for some time, or maybe I'd finally had enough and these new words just erupted from me.

"I'm going to change! I mean it! I'm going to change!" The words startled me. I looked at myself in the mirror. A pale, gaunt face with red-rimmed eyes and a sad mouth stared back. I knew my face so well, yet this face seemed like a stranger's. I examined myself as though I were looking at someone I didn't know. Who was this person? I felt a rush of compassion and an urge to help. It was not a feeling of pity but a genuine desire to help him out of the hole into which he'd fallen.

No more feeling sorry for myself, I vowed. The face in the mirror nodded solemnly. No more skipping therapy. No more skipping pills. No more skipping meals or classes. No more. . . .

There was a knock at the door. I opened it and there was the guy who'd showed me his baggie of pot that morning.

"Ready?" he asked, grinning.

I was definitely ready, but not for that. It would have been so easy to try it just once to escape, even temporarily from what I knew would be a grueling battle back. I wasn't sure I could do it. I didn't know if saving myself was even worth attempting. I thought of Brett's sneer and the whispers of, "Is he gay?" and the look of horror on the girl's face when she glimpsed me doing my therapy. I remembered the face in the mirror, looking and waiting—for this?

"Never mind," I told him. "You go ahead. I can't risk hurting myself."

His face fell. "Okay," he said with a shrug.

This was the first challenge to my new resolve, and I'd mastered it. Yes! Now, I had to take the next steps. I knew I had to make some drastic changes. I grabbed a notebook and a pen and turned to a clean page. I settled myself on the sofa and made a list: Ways to improve myself. What did I want? I wanted to play basketball, and I wanted to play it well. I wanted to be able to walk to my classes again. I wanted to go to classes and bring home a report card I'd be proud to show my parents. I wanted friends and a girlfriend. I looked at my watch. The time it showed didn't register with me because that time didn't matter. I knew deep inside my soul that my time was now.

Chapter 19
Getting a Huge Weight Off My Chest

When the alarm clock rang the next morning, something felt different. It took a minute to realize what it was. Then I remembered. Today was the day I would begin challenging myself to overcome my doubts, defeat cystic fibrosis and change the attitude that had been dragging me down.

I was not going to be the same self-pitying guy who had isolated himself from the world. It was going to be the biggest challenge of my life and I wasn't sure I could pull it off. Recovering from the hole I'd put myself in was not going to be easy. I immediately went back on my meds and began doing my therapy once, and sometimes twice, a day. I was still coughing and spitting up phlegm, but my stamina improved after just a few weeks. I was learning to control my emotions and was no longer angry at myself. I focused every bit of my energy on doing whatever it took to get better.

The following quarter I signed up for advanced weightlifting. I didn't need that class to graduate, and I wasn't taking it to help me through school. I was taking it to help me get through life.

Since entering college, I'd despised the way my body looked. I had bony arms and a skinny chest. My legs were like twigs. I was so embarrassed about my body that I refused to go to the university's swimming pool because I didn't want anyone to see how scrawny I was. I knew the guys would be shedding their shirts and catching the rays, so instead of going to the pool I'd tell my friends I had to do homework, or that my medicine made me too sensitive to the sun. When I played basketball and the teams were split into "shirts" and "skins," I sat. I didn't want girls to see how skinny I was.

On the first day of advanced weightlifting, I nervously entered the gym. My first observation gave me no encouragement at all. Many who'd signed up were obviously on the football team. Some of them were bigger than my car. I was afraid they might accidentally trample me. I did see with relief that my fraternity brother, Greg Green, was in the class, too, and looked as uneasy as I felt, which made me feel better. Suddenly someone bellowed, "Everyone quiet!"

Coach Mervos had entered the room. He was just five-foot-six but had forearms that looked like they could bend lead. "Everyone! Sit down and shut up!" he hollered. I figured that this was what prison or boot camp was like.

"I have three rules in my class," the coach said, eyeing us as though we were serving life sentences for murder. "First, no excuses if you're late. If you are tardy, you'll do a mile lap around the track. If you're late again, I'll double it. If you're late again, you fail.

"Second rule: You have to be here for every class. If you miss a day, you run the track. If you miss another day, you'll run farther. Miss three days…"

I knew where this was going.

"… and you fail. My third rule is everyone must participate. One person will count each day when we do push-ups. If he loses count, the whole class starts over. If you can't finish, you'll start over. Is this clear?"

"Yes, sir," we chimed in unison. My mouth said yes, but my brain was objecting. What was I getting myself into?

Next, Coach Mervos handed out disclaimer forms, which asked us to list any health problems. Not long ago, I would have written, "I have cystic fibrosis." on it. But today, I wrote "none." I'd have no excuse for not excelling.

Coach Mervos then said he would group us based on how much weight we could lift. Greg lifted about 175 pounds. I had a hunch I wouldn't be in his group. I'd never lifted weights, unless you counted my algebra book. I did know how to lift a 45-pound barbell from watching Josh when we were freshmen.

As Coach Mervos watched, I lifted 45 pounds. Then 65, 85 and then 105 pounds. I couldn't quite lift 115, but felt good with what I was able to lift. Then I saw that quite a few of the girls in the class could lift that much, too. I was humbled, and wondered, again, whether I was making a mistake.

Coach Mervos told me that by the time the ten-week class ended, he'd like me to be able to lift 155 pounds. I decided I'd reach for 165. It would be the first time I walked onto the UGA campus with a determination to exceed someone else's expectation of my abilities.

I went to a sporting goods store and bought workout gloves, Spandex shorts and some T-shirts. I wanted to look the part of a weightlifter, and the clothes gave me an extra boost of confidence. Those gloves got a lot of use. I lifted weights every day of class. I did pull-ups, push-ups, dips, curls and everything else Coach Mervos ordered. He always demanded more, and I realized I thrived on that challenge. Some days, I'd crawl out of class feeling like a jellyfish—wobbly and limp—but I didn't quit. Sometimes, I even went to the gym on weekends. If Coach Mervos said to do 10 sets, I'd do 11. If he called for 12 reps, I did 13. For the first time in a very long time, I was driven to succeed.

I would love to say that everything went smoothly—that I bulked up and everyone admired me. But it wasn't quite that easy, of course. One afternoon, a bunch of us were watching a baseball game on TV at the fraternity house. Brian—a fraternity brother and diehard weightlifter—glanced at me and grimaced.

"Andy," he said, "you really shouldn't roll up your sleeves like that until you get some muscles."

Everyone looked at my arms and I knew what they were thinking— scrawny. The guys chuckled, which reminded me of their reaction when Brett mocked me not that long ago. A few weeks prior, I might have stormed from the room. Though my pride was wounded, this time I just bit my lip and didn't say anything. Brian's comment made me realize I'd have to keep working to see results, and since that day, I've never rolled up my sleeves. Later, when someone commented that I was bulking up, I shrugged and said my shirt was tight.

Another goal I set was to be able to walk to classes without sounding and feeling like I had emphysema. I didn't share this goal with anyone, because I didn't want them to know I was exhausted walking, even after a quarter of a mile. I had often begged rides from my fraternity brothers, saying I hurt my leg or had to be in class early. I didn't want to admit how weak I was. I had even looked into taking what was called the "disability bus." A woman at the clinic told me it stopped right by the fraternity house. It seemed like a good idea— until I saw the girl.

From a distance, I watched the bus pull into the parking lot. A girl in a wheelchair using her mouth to guide the controls for her chair maneuvered onto the bus. She may have appeared disabled, but emotionally she was far stronger than I was. She was getting where she had to go. I realized then that my handicap was all in my head. I called it an *Andy-cap*. After seeing how courageously she handled herself, I knew I couldn't ask for a ride on her bus. After all, I had the ability to walk. I just lacked the mental strength to do it. That had to change.

The only way to get to class on time was to leave at least 15 minutes early. That way, I could take breaks to catch my breath, cough or spit up chunks of phlegm. Every day I walked, and every day I coughed and huffed and puffed. Friends would see me and offer to give me rides, but I always declined. They may have thought I was being rude—and maybe I should have explained my goal—but I was so unsure of whether I'd make it that I didn't want to tell anyone in case I failed.

By the end of the quarter, I could walk to class without gasping. I looked better from all the weightlifting, and I felt better, too. I was doing my therapy every day and taking all my medications. I began eating better, as well. Not that I wouldn't rather live on Shoney's strawberry pies, but I knew if I was going to get strong and stay that way, I needed to put high-test fuel in the engine. The better I felt, the happier I was.

At our last weightlifting class, it was time to examine our progress. There was only one way to measure success—how much weight could we lift compared to ten weeks earlier. I knew I looked better, but I remembered Brian's remark and worried that maybe I hadn't improved as much as I thought. That day, I lifted weights of different sizes, including 155 pounds, the goal Coach Mervos had set for me. I brought the weight to my chest and heaved it back onto the bar. I was sweating, but I'd done it. I'd reached that goal. Now I needed another. I asked for another fifteen pounds on the bar.

"Are you sure?" said the guy who was spotting me. I knew I looked exhausted. I was panting from the exertion, and my forehead and chest were damp with sweat, but my spirit was rejuvenated.

"Yup," I said, "put it on there."

I settled myself on the bench, took a few deep breaths and closed my eyes to gather my energy. I slowly counted to three and lifted. I lowered the bar to my chest and put everything I had into lifting it. I thought about all the people who doubted me. As I lifted the weight, I pushed them and their negativity up and away. For all that was balanced on the bar, it was surprisingly light. I'd exceeded my personal goal by lifting one-hundred-seventy pounds.

At the end of class, Coach Mervos went around the room and asked everyone to state their starting weight, his goal and their goal. When he said "Andy Lipman," I replied proudly, "One-hundred-seventy pounds." Greg gave me a respectful smile. That was something I hadn't seen in a long, long time.

I thought about the muscular guy whose picture once hung in my doctor's office. As an eight-year-old, I hoped that someday I could look like him. Now I was slowly turning into him.

I felt so happy I practically skipped home. I called Aunt Susie that night to tell her about the 170 pounds and together we rejoiced at my accomplishment. Looking back, however, the bigger accomplishment was the change in my attitude.

My health was improving. I faithfully took the antibiotics my doctor prescribed. After several weeks of hard work, my phlegm was clear again and I returned to sleeping on my loft. My grades improved that quarter, along with my attendance. I understood more of the lectures, and they became more interesting. I got into a routine I liked—classes in the morning, gym in the afternoon, and the library at night.

My fraternity brothers noticed these changes, or maybe it was just that I didn't feel so defensive and self-pitying. I stopped feeling sorry for myself, and I didn't expect anyone else to feel sorry for me, either. I wanted friendship and company. I wanted to be treated like one of them, and that meant not distancing myself. I'd stopped hiding in my room and when someone asked if I wanted to get something to eat or go to a movie, I swallowed my fears that they were asking only because they pitied me. The more I said yes, the less hesitancy I had about making friends, and the more likely they were to invite me again.

I made a special effort with Josh. I had thrown his friendship away while I was depressed and I know he noticed. He had even called my mom several times, fearing that my life was in danger. Josh and I now spent many days together at the gym and the library.

I was thrilled when, later that year, I was elected vice president of TEP and became the fraternity's athletic chairman and pledge trainer. If that wasn't enough of a turnaround, the biggest surprise was that during my senior year, I was named "most congenial brother," despite those bitter confrontations my sophomore and junior years. That award meant everything to me. It made me realize that my newfound strengths weren't going unnoticed by the people who saw me every day and knew me best. I was making more time for my friends and having more intimate conversations. As a result, they saw me as a person they wanted to represent them. I felt really good about all this, but there was still one score to settle.

Chapter 20
Picking My Moment

To the other five guys who played basketball that day, it was probably just another pick-up game—a way to get some exercise, blow off steam and hang out. To me, though, it was a shot at redemption.

I hadn't planned to play that afternoon. What I really wanted was a shower and a big glass of cool water because I'd been working out at the gym. I was exhausted, but infused with a peaceful feeling that almost always comes after pushing myself physically. I flopped down on the sofa by the basketball court, content to sun myself and watch my fraternity brothers vie for baskets.

I didn't expect them to ask me to play. I couldn't forget the humiliation I'd felt when Brett plowed me over and then mockingly scraped me off the asphalt like curbside litter. I wondered if they remembered the incident as keenly as I did.

Three-on-three basketball can't be played with just five guys, and when one guy gasped that he'd had enough and headed inside, everyone on the court looked to me. In those few months I'd developed some pride and a much stronger upper body. I was willing to play, not only to prove that I could, but also because I had a score to settle. One of the players on the other team was Brett. This was my chance to set the record straight, and my opponents that day were Brett and cystic fibrosis.

Despite my workout before the game, I felt energized and lively as soon as the game began. I was alert and quick, grabbing the ball and shooting. Sometimes I made the basket and sometimes I missed, but I never felt wheezy. I moved with the confidence and vigor I'd been lacking the last time.

The game was in its final minutes when Brett got the ball.

"Shoot!" someone yelled.

He never got the chance. As he aimed the ball, a feisty five-foot-eight inch, 150-pound kid slammed into him. Brett's feet flew out from under him and he fell onto the unforgiving asphalt. He looked stunned, especially as my teammate sank a jump shot with the ball he'd held just seconds before.

Take that, I thought, as I glared down at him. *No one's ever knocking me down, again.*

Brett raised his hand to me, implying that he wanted me to pull him up, but I ignored the unspoken request.

"Get your own self up," I muttered as I walked away and wiped my hands on my shorts. For the first time in a long time, I was standing up for myself.

I don't remember who won the game. It doesn't really matter. I won because I showed that I wouldn't let cystic fibrosis—or anyone—get the best of me. When we finished, we all gave each other high-fives, a TEP tradition. Brett and I slapped our sweaty palms together, and he mentioned that I looked like I'd been working out. I knew that was his way of apologizing. I found myself feeling a flash of appreciation for his motivating me out of my funk. His disparaging comments ultimately helped turn me around.

I ambled through the backdoor and directly to my room so no one would think that this basketball game was a big deal, but as soon as I shut the door, I cranked up "Eye of the Tiger," ripped off my T-shirt and danced around like a tourist at Mardi Gras.

As I danced, I caught a glimpse of myself in the mirror. For the first time in a long time, I was pleased with what I saw. Grinning back at me was a slightly red-faced, slightly breathless guy with strong arms and a muscular chest, and he was radiating an unmistakable confidence. It was that confidence that finally brought me what I longed for—a girlfriend.

I first saw Bryna from the Tau Epsilon Phi basketball court. I was twenty-one, shirtless and shooting baskets, but still too intimidated to strike up a conversation with someone so pretty and effervescent. She was there to deliver cookies to some of her friends at the fraternity house.

When I ran into her several months later at a college bar, we chatted about Michael Jordan. I was impressed. Never before had I talked to a girl about sports, and Bryna knew her stuff. I wanted to ask her for a date, but was still too intimidated. Instead, I told her that I'd make her a bet. I'd buy her dinner if Georgia lost to Alabama. I knew I had a chance because our team was pretty bad that year. For the first—and only—time, I hoped my Bulldogs would lose. They did, and we had our first date.

Bryna and I dated for a little over a year. She was not Jewish, but that wasn't a big deal to me. Several of my fraternity brothers only dated Jewish women because they were thinking long-term. If the relationships got serious and led to marriage, procreation became an issue. Most of us wanted to raise our kids Jewish. Maybe I shouldn't use the term "us." I knew I probably couldn't have kids, so I didn't think it mattered who I dated. I just wanted a good person and, to be honest, I wasn't thinking about marriage.

Having a girlfriend was pretty awesome. First, I didn't feel like a third wheel when my fraternity brothers were hanging with their girlfriends and me. Second, I didn't have to find dates to functions. Finally, I had someone I really cared about. It was nice knowing that someone saw me for me, and not as a person with a life-threatening disease.

I began attending shows where Bryna displayed her artwork, and she watched me play softball and basketball. Bryna was also a UGA batgirl for the baseball team, so I got to watch my favorite pastime and support my girlfriend at the same time. It was a great relationship, except for one thing. I always thought the hardest questions in a relationship would be, "Do you love me?" and "Why do you have to watch *SportsCenter* every night?" Instead, it was "Why don't we ever talk about cystic fibrosis?"

It was a tough topic for me. Everything I knew about it was negative: I wasn't supposed to live past twenty-five, many kids with CF were frail and sickly, and it made me feel vulnerable—and scared. I preferred to talk about my friends, the fraternity, Bryna, my parents, my plans and anything else positive.

Bryna knew I had cystic fibrosis because one of her friends told her. I wish I had been the one to tell her, because I probably could have found a way to make CF sound less than it is. The first time we talked in any depth about CF, she began to cry, which made me feel terrible. I felt inadequate and guilty for bringing sadness to someone I loved. She also pitied me, which didn't help. I didn't want her pity. I wanted support. I wanted her to say, "Andy, I'm not worried. I know you'll defy the odds." In retrospect, we shouldn't have had the conversation on the phone. It was too impersonal and I couldn't accurately gauge her reaction. Also, I couldn't hug her because we were miles apart. We had the CF conversation plenty of times, but she was always the one to bring it up. She had a lot of questions, but because I was so reluctant to discuss it, she too became edgy whenever the subject arose.

When we broke up, it didn't have anything to do with CF. It was just time for us to look elsewhere. The day we decided we'd stop seeing each other was also the day Bryna told me she'd been reading about cystic fibrosis and knew more than I did. I guess she told me because she wanted me to know how deep her feelings were for me.

Looking back, I wish I'd been more open about CF with Bryna. I just didn't know how. I considered it something personal that affected just me, and maybe my parents. I did my best to keep it from having any role in my friendships, because I didn't want it to overshadow anything else about me. But that's like saying the fact that I'm Jewish is something to hide, or that I'm a sports junkie is something no one should know. Not that that would have been possible, anyway. Those things are all part of who I am, and to deny any of them is to give a false picture of myself. It's not like I can do anything to get rid of CF, but that doesn't mean it has to rule my life. Trying to find the right balance for cystic fibrosis has never been easy, especially with a girlfriend in the picture.

I wrestled with those same issues when I began dating a girl named Stephanie. She was a sister of the D Phi E sorority, one of the two Jewish sororities on campus. My mom was also a sister and, coincidently, the national charity of D Phi E was the Cystic Fibrosis Foundation.

The first time Stephanie and I spent any time together was at the supermarket. It takes a pretty amazing woman to get me to go to the grocery store—especially on a Saturday at midnight. We discovered we had a lot of similar interests and began to date a few months before my graduation.

I should have learned something about dealing with cystic fibrosis from my relationship with Bryna, but I made many of the same mistakes again. The biggest was sidestepping the topic for so long that someone else told Stephanie. Of course she was upset, but it was hard to determine if she was upset because of what she'd heard about CF or because I hadn't been trusting and open enough to tell her myself. I hadn't wanted to tell her because I was afraid she would have the same reaction as Bryna, and I wasn't eager to deal with more tears.

We talked over the phone, which I vowed I wouldn't do again when it came to such a heavy topic, and yes, Stephanie cried. What I didn't realize then was that she was crying because she was concerned about me. Come to think of it, my mom is the same way.

I thought the conversation with Stephanie would be the first and last we'd have about CF. Then we could continue with a "normal" relationship that involved fraternity and sorority parties, spring break and movies. Stephanie kept bringing it up though, and I kept dodging her questions. Sometimes I'd fake being asleep or claim I was too tired to talk. Sometimes I'd even use CF as an excuse not to talk about CF, saying I wasn't feeling well enough. That really upset her.

It came down to this: despite my repeated successes in overcoming the limitations imposed by CF, I couldn't think of anything positive to say about a potentially fatal disease, and if I couldn't think of something positive, I wasn't going to say anything. I wasn't willing to admit I was afraid that if she knew too much about CF, she'd see how vulnerable I was or treat me differently. I wanted her to admire and respect and adore me. I thought if she knew the truth, she'd run.

That may have sounded like a reasonable plan, but it didn't work, thank goodness. A relationship where there's a big snarling monster both people have to tiptoe around can't thrive. So, one night I took the plunge and poured out to Stephanie everything I'd kept bottled up inside.

I told her I probably couldn't have children. I told her how I reacted to the encyclopedia article and how my parents feared for my health. I even told her about the hardest time of my life—those many months when I sank so low that I wanted to die. I confessed that I'd hidden my therapy machine and medicines the first time she came over. I told her how many people were unnerved by CF and how sometimes it unnerved even me. We talked for hours . . . or, I should say, unlike most of our conversations, I talked and she listened. I cried that night like I cried during those nights in my room when I felt so isolated. I was afraid that once Stephanie knew the true me, she'd be out the door. But she wasn't.

In fact, the opposite happened. The honesty helped bind us. It cleared the air, and improved the trust and openness between us. Our relationship changed for the better, and I changed, too. I showed Stephanie my therapy machine and medicines and told her when I had doctor appointments. It was awkward at first, but the more I talked about these things that were part of my life, the easier it got for both of us. The topic was no longer taboo, so she relaxed, which made me more comfortable talking to her. One day, I even shared with her my dream of defeating CF forever. I knew she'd nod and give me a hug, which was just what I needed.

Sometimes I wondered if she ever thought, "Why am I with this guy?" It took me a while to figure out that she loved me as much as I loved her, and CF just happened to be part of the Andy Lipman deluxe package. Stephanie helped me realize I didn't have to hide cystic fibrosis from anyone, and I didn't have to hide from CF.

Stephanie and I dated for about two years. Our breakup had less to do with distance—she moved back to her hometown of Dallas to become a kindergarten teacher—than fear. My fear. I was afraid to make a commitment to someone without being sure I could fulfill it. Though I was healthy and optimistic about my future, when I got to thinking about us, I realized I couldn't guarantee her a long life together. I couldn't guarantee we'd be able to have children, and I knew from the career she'd chosen that kids were very important to her.

I loved Stephanie and I regret that my low self-esteem caused us to break up. But I am grateful that we were able to maintain a friendship. For a long time, there was no one who knew me as intimately as she did, and she became a great person to provide support and advice—even on dating. I did the same for her. We'd be on the phone and I'd ask, "Do you think I should bring up CF on the second date or the third?" She'd say, "Just wait until there's a point when it fits into the conversation."

"Good idea," I'd say. Because, "So, you want dessert? And, oh, I have CF," might not be the best way to go.

Stephanie eventually got married and has two beautiful children. She still lives in Dallas. Bryna is back in Athens working at the University of Georgia. I rarely hear from her, but Stephanie and I keep up more regularly.

The bright side was—though I'd broken up with two great girls—I realized that I could be in a long-term relationship and that I could be more open about my cystic fibrosis. This was another step I had needed to take to improve my self-esteem.

Chapter 21
CF Attacks . . . But not in the Lungs

Late in my senior year, I was disappointed to learn I needed another year of school to graduate. Due to academic slippage as a sophomore, I would be the last of my pledge class to graduate. Thank goodness for Haim (pronounced Hi-um) Cohen. He was my roommate that summer and quite possibly the best roommate I ever had. Haim was from Miami and was enthusiastic about everything.

"Haim, you want to go eat?" I'd ask.

He'd say he wanted steak, but he wouldn't just say the word "steak." Several adjectives preceded it like "Tasty, juicy, and succulent."

"Haim, you want to work out?"

"I'm going to embarrass everyone else in the gym. I'm going to crank it today. Yeah, man, I'm going to rip some sets off today." He'd always have me in hysterics.

We both loved sports, food and exercise, and got along like brothers— or how I assumed brothers would get along. Not having one, I couldn't really say, but anyone who's as close to his brother as Haim and I were is lucky.

Early in our relationship, Haim witnessed one of the most frightening experiences of my life. Fortunately, for me, he wasn't just a bystander, but someone who took charge of the situation. I don't know what would have happened if he hadn't.

Haim was the quarterback of our pledge football team, and I was one of the wide receivers, though I never played a down in the Alpha Epsilon PI/ TEP game. He used to tell me the only good thing about my hands was that I never dropped the cup of water I handed him from the sidelines. I used to tell him that the great thing about him was that he was free of prejudice; he threw the ball to both our teammates and our opponents.

What Haim lacked on the gridiron, he made up for in the kitchen. This guy could cook. He made dinner almost every night, and I did the dishes. It was like living with my mom, but without her interrogations. Haim's cooking skills didn't rub off on me, but his diligence did. The summer of 1995, after our senior year, he studied at least four hours every night for the medical school admission test. He was taking classes during the day, working out in the afternoons and studying late into the night. Plus, like me, he was involved in a long-distance relationship. His girlfriend was spending the summer in Atlanta on an internship.

Bryna was my girlfriend then and she was studying in Europe. Most of my friends had left, too. Josh and another close friend, Will Shields, had graduated, so I was really feeling lonely. But Haim more than made up for their absences. We talked about the difficulties of long-distance relationships, and we debated endlessly about who was a better athlete. We lifted weights together at least once a week, and we ate like a famine was looming.

Haim grew up in an observant Jewish family, and while my upbringing was less strict, we were compatible. My family liked him, too. Whenever my dad came to visit, he'd take us to the grocery store and load food into the cart. I'd tell my dad we had enough, but Haim would give me a look that shut me up, and he'd drop in another armful or two. Haim was notorious around our fraternity house as a world-class eater. Of course, I was no slouch either.

A lot of people with cystic fibrosis are thin because their higher-than-average metabolism burns a lot of extra calories. They're constantly worried about trying to gain weight, and usually can't. That's not a problem for me. Just to win a bet, I once ate two twelve-inch Little Caesar's pizzas and an order of breadsticks and washed it all down with a large Coke.

That summer, we planned a July Fourth barbecue. Naturally, Haim was going to do the honors at the grill. I couldn't wait. He made the most amazing ribs and chicken.

To get ready for the feast, I popped three Pancrease pills, the enzymes that helped me digest fat. The more I planned to eat, the more pills I'd have to take. I'd been taking those pills for as long as I could remember. This time, though, I seriously underestimated how much I'd eat. I devoured 10 ribs, four pieces of chicken, some rice and some corn. The food smelled so good, and it just kept coming. We were all kicking back, reminiscing about college and speculating about where we'd be in 10 years. I didn't really think about what I was eating.

I woke up the next morning with a mild stomach-ache. The pain was somewhat dull. I sat on the toilet for half an hour, but I couldn't go. Darn. I went to class anyway. Summer school was starting, and I wanted to make a good impression. However, as the day progressed, the pain got worse. Just sitting in class was painful. I remembered the throbbing hurt all too well. When I was in grade school, there was an occasion where my mom had to give me an enema every day for a full week. No way was I going through that again.

After my last class, I went straight to the student health center. That's how desperate I was. The joke around campus was that whether you were suffering a heart attack or a sore throat, you'd get the same treatment—a prescription for amoxicillin and instructions to take it easy.

I told the doctor my problem and that I had CF. I could see in his eyes that he was unnerved. I imagined him thinking: "Cystic fibrosis! Hmm . . . Now what did we learn in medical school about CF? Aha! Where's that amoxicillin?" He told me I ate too much—well, I knew that!—and to lie on my side. He pulled a plastic glove onto his hand, then stuck his hand into my rectum and removed the feces stuck inside me. Then he gave me an enema to clean out whatever was left.

It sounds gross, and it was. When he was done, I couldn't look him in the eye, but I felt so much better. There was just a slight pain in my stomach, but the doctor said it was normal. I swore to myself that no matter how tantalizing the food looked, I'd never, ever eat like that again.

When I got home, I told Haim about my big adventure, though I spared him some of the details. I felt so much better that I worked out and then studied. It was a tough and embarrassing day, but I felt good because I'd taken care of my health on my own. My mom tends to be overprotective, but this experience proved to me that I was capable of watching out for my own health. I was pretty proud of myself.

All of that changed the next morning. I woke up with a more intense pain than the day before. I struggled through my morning classes and that afternoon, I went back to the health center. The doctor I'd seen the day before wasn't there, but a nurse gave me several enemas to release the stool blockage. She asked if the pain had stopped. I told her it had, but I was lying. Honestly, I just wanted to get the heck out of there. Being naked—intensely naked—in front of a nurse and then having her administer enemas might show up on somebody's radar as a bizarre fantasy, but for me, it was pure horror. I'd had enough.

I staggered home and fell into bed. I couldn't sleep and I didn't know how to ease the pain. I didn't want to go through the whole humiliating experience again at a hospital, and I definitely did not want to call my folks. I was an adult and I could take care of myself . . . at least I thought I could.

When Haim got home, he knew something was wrong, though I insisted I was fine. He made stir-fry and brought it to my room, but I couldn't eat more than a few bites. When he saw I wasn't eating, he looked at me warily.

"I ate earlier," I lied.

My parents called half an hour later to say goodbye before leaving for Israel the next day. Mom suspected something was wrong. I didn't want her to know how terrible I felt because then they'd rush to see me and cancel their trip. I didn't want to mess up their plans. I assured her I was fine, and she seemed persuaded. After we hung up, I thought about my situation: Let's say I don't feel

THE DRIVE AT 35

better tomorrow. My folks are overseas. My doctor is several hundred miles away and I don't have a doctor in town who knows anything about me. What the heck would I do?

When the phone rang again, Haim grabbed it. "Andy has a terrible stomach ache," I heard him say, "Since Monday." Mom must've asked him if he thought they should come because my buddy, the guy who was studying to be a doctor said, "It's probably a good idea."

My parents arrived several hours later, and I realized how desperately I needed their help. Luckily for me, they're veterans when it comes to dealing with my medical emergencies. Paramedics have nothing on my folks. They immediately called Dr. Boat and told him my whole sorry story. He instructed me to drink a jug of a liquid called Golytely, the stuff stomach surgery patients drink before their operation.

At that point, I was all for it. Bring on the medical cocktail. This couldn't be any worse than the enemas. At least that's what I thought. I wouldn't even have to get undressed. Turned out Golytely was the worst tasting stuff I've ever swallowed. It could be used for enemy torture. It was clear, but viscous, like mineral oil, and tasted like week-old milk. I managed to choke down five glasses.

"I can't drink anymore," I sobbed. "I'm going to throw up."

Mom looked just as upset as I felt, but she knew the situation was serious. Drink it, she urged, or we'll have to take you to the hospital.

"Okay," I said. "Let's go."

I think that was the only time I didn't offer a word of objection when my folks wanted to take me to see a doctor. I couldn't stop crying, and was doubled over in pain. My parents, one on each side, practically carried me into the car. I vividly remember the look of terror on Haim's face as my parents guided me out.

At St. Mary's Hospital, Mom maneuvered me into a wheelchair and we waited in the emergency room. After what seemed like an eternity, a nurse called my name. I was wheeled into a room where a doctor asked me a long list of questions, and hooked me up to an IV to ease my pain. I don't remember much, thank goodness, but I do recall the bright lights and the sensation of having my pants unzipped and pulled off my legs. Here we go again with the enemas. At least I didn't have to look anyone in the eye. Eventually, I was cleaned out. Exhausted, I was sent home with orders to always match my enzyme intake to my food intake. It was definitely a lesson that stuck. No pun intended.

My condition, I later learned from reading medical books, was called distal intestinal obstruction syndrome, or DIOS. It's pretty common among people with cystic fibrosis. I remembered from Spanish class that "Dios" means God. My experience was pretty ungodly, I'd say.

I spent five days in Atlanta with my folks recuperating. The pain was gone, but so was my energy. I was wiped out, physically and emotionally. On the fifth day, my dad drove me back to school and urged me to take it easy. Then he and Mom went on their trip to Israel and Europe. Haim was glad to see me and suggested I go to the gym to get my strength back.

I shook my head in frustration. "I can't," I told him, recounting the long tale of enemas, pain and humiliation.

"C'mon, man. Don't be lazy," he said. That was all I needed to hear. Me? Lazy? Not a chance.

I worked out that day for the first time in more than a week, and I worked out the rest of the week, too. I got back into the groove of studying, spending three or four hours a night on my classes. It shouldn't be any big surprise that my grades improved. In fact, I made all "A's" that quarter. Haim's impressive study habits rubbed off on me. So did his dedication to fitness. By the end of the summer, I was in the best shape I'd ever been.

It was fitting the DIOS happened when I lived with Haim. He ended up becoming a podiatrist, and practices in Cincinnati, Ohio—the same city where Dr. Boat now practices. I am able to stay with Haim and his family any time I need.

As fall rolled around, and the rest of the students began arriving for the new school year, I realized I'd had a heck of a summer. I'd fought DIOS in one of the toughest CF battles I'd ever had, and I realized that whatever punches cystic fibrosis threw at me, I could face them. I'd stared down my opponent, and I was still standing. Not only that, I looked pretty darn good in the ring.

The following year, I graduated from the University of Georgia with my BBA. While this academic milestone was important in my life, it paled to the significance of beating cystic fibrosis the prior summer. July 4, 1995, was truly an Independence Day for me. Cystic fibrosis didn't control my life any more, and I knew I could beat it if I put my mind to it. I had plans for the next July 4th, too—a little something to keep CF on the run.

I was nearly twenty-two when I decided it was time. My attitude was different. I could do things I once didn't believe I could. That meant going after the big prize. I called Uncle Bobby and told him: "I'm going to put on that T-shirt."

He knew exactly what I meant.

"We'll see," he said. "You've said that before. Why should this time be any different?"

I paused. "Because I want it. I really want it. See you on the Fourth."

Aunt Susie got on the phone.

"Andy, honey," she said, "you know you don't have to run the whole thing, or any of it. You can walk and get that T-shirt. That's okay, too."

"If I'm going to enter the Peachtree Road Race, I'm going to run it," I said, annoyed that she'd be so quick to cut her nephew a break. "I don't do things half-way."

Nine years before, I'd quit on the dream. I had other plans this time around. This year I was going to conquer the 6.2-mile monster.

A soon as the race applications appeared in the Atlanta newspaper, I filled one out and mailed it. I could see myself crossing the finish line and my uncle picking me up on his shoulders and parading me around. Friends would be cheering my victory, and I might be sweaty and tired, but I'd wear my new T-shirt—the one I earned with every step—to breakfast that morning.

It was a good fantasy, but I had a way to go to make it a reality. I hadn't even begun to train for the race. I figured that when I got my number, it would be the green light I needed to start working toward this goal.

An envelope from the race people arrived about a month later. I decided I'd hang the race number it contained on my bulletin board to motivate me. But there was no race number inside. Instead, there was a form letter. My application had been rejected, because I forgot to send a picture ID. I was dumbfounded.

I should have blamed myself for not reading the application carefully enough. Instead, I vented all my rage on my mom. "Why didn't you tell me I needed to send a picture ID?" I demanded.

"Andy, I can't do everything. You filled out the application. You should have read it more carefully."

That July 4th, my uncle Bobby was in his usual fine form. "Did you see me on TV?" he gloated. "How did I look? I'm glad you almost ran it again this year."

After I hung up the phone, I thought of what I should have said: "I almost run it every year."

Chapter 22
A Reason to Run

Nearly a year after the racing number fiasco, I still had stuff from my college apartment in boxes. I figured my baseball cards, all fifty thousand of them, must be in there somewhere, so on a Saturday when there was nothing on TV, I began digging through the boxes. Something I found amid the Nerf basketball net and baseball caps restored my drive to run the Peachtree.

It was a bookmark shaped like a tennis racket. I'd forgotten that I saved it, but I remembered exactly when I got it. I was about seventeen and helping at my dad's company party. Becky Decker, his secretary, wished me a happy birthday and told me she'd heard I'd made the school's tennis team. The bookmark, she said, would remind me to do my best at school and tennis. I didn't know Becky all that well, but from my dad I knew that Becky was one of the most thoughtful people around. The fact that she not only remembered my birthday, but also my interests, said a lot about her.

A few years later, when I was in college, my mother told me Becky had cancer. How could that be? I was the one with the incurable disease; she was a lively person who lit up any room she entered. I was very sad when she died a few months later. My dad gave a eulogy at her funeral. He framed a poem he wrote about her and hung it in the conference room at his office.

I remembered what Becky said when she gave me the bookmark: ". . . do your best. . . ." Had I really done my best? Not when it came to the Peachtree Road Race. I dialed Bobby's number, my speed increasing with each digit I punched, before I could change my mind.

When he heard my recurring, "I'm going to run the Peachtree" pledge, he chuckled. "You're kidding, right?" Same old Bobby.

"Let's pretend I'm not," I said. "I want your help."

"Okay," he said. "Start with running once a week. Run for time, not distance. Build your stamina. Don't worry how far or how fast. Just go. And run on the street. Don't use a treadmill; it won't help you learn how to handle hills."

I began training in January 1997, a good six months before the race. On a chilly Saturday morning, I walked outside, stretched a little and set off at a slow jog. God, it felt good to be running again. My feet hit the street rhythmically and the air was crisp and fresh.

A quarter-mile from home I was slammed by a severe coughing attack. I doubled over, spitting thick gobs of phlegm into the street. When the attack subsided, I could barely breathe. I couldn't run anymore. I stopped and limped a few feet toward home. Wrenched by another coughing fit, I heaved up more phlegm. I was soaked in sweat. To make matters worse, I was having shin splints and my legs were killing me. I sat on the side of the street and then slowly made my way home. Damn cystic fibrosis!

I began training every other day, and stretched more to avoid the shin splints. When I could run a quarter-mile, I pushed the distance to a half-mile then a mile. I was one-sixth of the way there. I was still coughing badly sometimes, but every time I called Bobby to update him on my progress, I was a little more confident.

"You're on your way," he said at the end of one of those calls.

That's as close as Bobby gets to praise, and hearing it, I figured he believed in me. A few weeks later, I knew it for a fact. He'd purchased a membership for me in the Atlanta Track Club, whose members have an edge in being chosen for the race.

A week later, when the application for the race appeared in the paper, I filled it out and wrote my eighteen-dollar check. This time, I remembered to include a copy of my picture ID. After my last devastating experience, there's no way I would have forgotten that! Then I examined a dozen mailboxes in my neighborhood to see which had the earliest pickup, because the postmark can be critical in getting a number for the race.

Before I dropped the envelope down the mail chute, I prayed right there on the sidewalk: "Please, God, let my application go through. I've never wanted anything more than to run this race. I want Bobby's respect. I want to do this for Becky. Please." Somebody heard my prayer.

By spring, I was up to three miles as often as four times a week. Then in late May, I did something stupid. Though Bobby had told me not to run on the treadmill, one night I was watching a movie on TV while jogging barefoot on the treadmill. I was surprised to see I'd covered more than four miles. Just two more would be the distance of the Peachtree. Could I do it? I've never met a challenge I didn't like. I stopped when I hit seven miles.

The next morning was payback for jogging barefoot. What a moron! I couldn't bend my knees. I worked at Enterprise Rent-A-Car then, which required a lot of walking. Unfortunately, I could barely hobble. I had to wear a brace on each knee when I played outfield on my softball team. I even had to take myself out of a game because the pain was so intense. I'd ice my knees every night and wake up each morning in more pain.

I didn't go to see a doctor, though that probably would have been a very good idea. I've got nothing against doctors, but after spending so much time with them as a sick kid, these days, I honestly prefer to let them have time with other patients.

I'm sure a doctor would have warned me to take a breather from running for a few weeks, but I knew that if I gave up, I'd never be ready for the race I'd set my heart on. Two weeks later, despite the injury, I forced myself to run and felt okay. I'm finally over the Peachtree hex, I told myself proudly. I wiped the sweat from my face and in an instant saw my hand was smeared with red. My nose was gushing blood so badly I had to peel off my T-shirt and use it to stop the bleeding. My knees were swollen. Was this God's way of telling me to give up on the race? The wrenched ankle. The application problem. Now this.

Full of pity for myself, I called Stephanie, whom I was still dating, to commiserate. Actually, I was supposed to call her earlier, but I was so preoccupied with the race that I'd forgotten. She was furious, and looking back, I can't blame her. She was on vacation and had canceled plans just to talk with me. Then I'd never called. Our argument escalated, and we broke up over the phone. I slammed down the receiver and cried. Stephanie was an important person in my life. She was the first person to get me to open up about cystic fibrosis and I'd disappointed her. I was madder at myself than at her.

Three weeks later, on the night of July 3rd, I was at Bobby's doorstep with my gym bag in one hand and my running shoes in the other. I wasn't sure I could finish the Peachtree. All I knew was I had to start. I thought of Becky, the bookmark, and her urging me to do my best.

After a massive spaghetti dinner, Bobby and I went to bed at ten o'clock. My alarm was set for 4:30 am, but I couldn't sleep. I must have, though, because Aunt Susie woke me up by rubbing my shoulder and saying, "Today's the day!"

The sky was still dark when we arrived at the starting area. The moon was out and the crickets were yielding to the first birds of the morning. I turned on my Walkman for some of the tunes I'd put on a tape to get me pumped: "Eye of the Tiger," "Jump" and "Welcome to the Jungle." I adjusted my knee braces—black and red, University of Georgia colors—and wrapped Becky's bookmark around my wrist, tucking it under my wristband. After the race, I framed it and hung it in my room as a source of inspiration. "I admire you, Becky," I whispered, "and my effort is in your honor."

Before I even crossed the starting line, I was sweating and my knees were sore. Bobby was trying to be supportive, but every time he said, "Relax, big boy. You're gonna be fine," I'd just get more stressed. So much was riding on this: the desire to prove myself to me and to my family, along with the memory of Becky and her heartbreaking fight against cancer.

I drew energy from the crowd. People were clapping and singing. Some held up signs with the names of family members and friends in the race. One man was wearing a shirt that said, "I had a heart attack one year ago, and here I am today." Everyone who passed him patted him on the back in support. Seeing the cheering along the sidelines, Bobby suggested, "Let the crowd take you to the finish line."

So off we went. I felt great at the one-mile mark. One-sixth of the way there. Knees fine, adrenaline good. Two mile mark: a third of the way there. A few coughs, but nothing serious.

At the two-and-a-half mark, I saw signs saying, "Go Bobby and Andy!" My parents, Susie, cousins Erin and Drew—and even Stephanie—were there cheering. Though there was no question we'd broken up, there she was. She knew how important that T-shirt was to me, and she hadn't forgotten. My folks took pictures as we ran because there was no way I was going to stop once I'd started.

Heartbreak Hill—halfway through, and the toughest part of the race—is a half-mile up, and it's where many of the twenty thousand runners walk or even quit. There were several times in the past when runners had heart attacks there, or even died, but I kept running. This race had become a one-on-one, me against cystic fibrosis. I felt a little winded, but I didn't dare stop. I coughed up some phlegm. I kept going. If CF couldn't stop me, Heartbreak Hill certainly couldn't.

Five miles. The end was in sight. I began waving my fist and clapping along with the crowd. With each step, I was closer to the finish line. I was on the verge of finishing a 10K run, and several years ago I couldn't even walk to class.

Six miles. My knees began to swell and the pain became intense. We entered Piedmont Park, and I had just a fifth of a mile to go. God, it hurt. But instead of quitting or walking, I did something Bobby warned me never to do. I sprinted to the finish line.

Like everyone else who completed the race, I received a 1997 Peachtree Road Race T-shirt. Bobby, who finished a few seconds behind me, got one too.

"Congratulations, big man," he said, sweaty and breathless, but smiling. "I'm proud of you. I knew you could do it."

I was proud that I'd finally earned his respect by following through on a promise I made nearly a decade ago. I felt such a huge sense of achievement. Finishing this race was something I never thought I could do—something just about everyone thought I couldn't do. It was exhilarating to prove that hard work really could beat the statistics.

We picked our way through the sweaty crowds of runners and supporters. It was nearly noon. My parents were both in tears. I hugged them both, which was out of character, but absolutely right.

I should explain that I never hug my dad. Since my first Little League tryout, we have an understanding that a handshake is as good as a hug. It was that way with my dad and his dad, too. On this day, however, we gripped each other and held on tight.

On the way home for much-needed showers, Bobby asked, "Are you satisfied now that you have your T-shirt?"

Yes and no, I thought. I was satisfied that I did the one thing I was never able to do. I'd run the race doctors never thought I could—the race I had doubts I could finish. On the other hand, I'm not one to stay satisfied for long. As soon as I accomplish something, I set a new goal. There's a sign in my office that says, "Success is a journey, not a destination." It keeps me striving, though I realize I sometimes don't take enough time to enjoy the victories along the way, like finishing a race I'd always dreamed of running.

There would have been nothing shameful about answering Bobby with "Yeah, I'm satisfied—for now." Instead, almost to spite myself, I raised the bar even higher. I told myself that I wouldn't wear this shirt until I ran my next Peachtree and earned another.

"I'll be back next year," I proudly announced.

True to my word, I was back the following year, and the year after that, and the year after that. In fact, every year since that first race I came back to Peachtree Road to satisfy my hunger for the T-shirt. The T-shirts began adding up and soon I had a drawer full, just like my uncle.

I loved wearing my Peachtree T-shirts, but the race was about a lot more than earning a shirt. It was about proving to myself that despite the odds, anything was possible. I proved that again a few years later through weight training.

I work out for an hour six mornings a week. Twice a week, I concentrate on each of three areas—chest, shoulders and back; biceps and triceps; and legs and abs. Also twice a week, I lift three sets with the barbell on my bench and 25 to 35 pounds per arm with dumbbells. I also run as the weather gets warmer.

The routine has changed my life. The exercise has probably saved it.

The hard work paid off in the weight room when, for the first time, I lifted 300 pounds on the flat bench.

Accomplishing athletic feats became a big part of my life. I only wish I could have shared them with my older sister.

Chapter 23

Meeting Wendy

My Aunt Susie remembers the tragedy like it was yesterday.

"I was 14 or 15 at the time," she said. "Your mother was pregnant with Wendy, and their dog, Lash, who in some ways was their first child, had just been killed by a car. I had been to visit Eva and Charles and I painted a huge mural of animals on the nursery wall in anticipation of Wendy's birth. Wendy was to be the first grandchild of both Eva's and Charles's families. I remember being in a coffee house in Jacksonville, Florida with friends, when I learned I was an aunt. I was so happy. Two weeks later, Wendy was gone. Nothing was really explained to me. It was a devastating loss for Eva and Charles. Two things about that time are indelible for me—the way Charles held Eva's hand in silence in the car the whole way to the funeral, and the tiny white casket we buried that day," Susie said. "Eva was a broken person. She was not the person you know as your mother. There was no life or laughter after the death of Wendy."

Growing up, I saw traces of mom's pain about Wendy's death. Every December, around the time of Wendy's birthday, my mom reminded me how lucky I was to be alive. I was a young boy then and was dealing with several traumatic secrets of my own. It angered me that my mom kept insinuating that I should feel blessed. With everything that I'd dealt with in my young life, I did not feel fortunate.

Three decades after Wendy's death, it was almost as if Wendy never existed. As far as I knew, there was nothing tangible in my parents' house to tell anyone they once had a daughter named Wendy, except for one hospital picture my mom kept tucked away. Aunt Susie said it was one of my mom's most precious possessions. I had never seen that snapshot, and I wasn't about to ask her for it. I wish she'd offered, but she never did.

I knew nothing of Wendy's existence, and I realized that after my parents died, there'd be no one left who remembered anything about her. I was at a point in my life where I wanted something from Wendy that I could see and touch, something that proved she had lived, however briefly.

Then I realized what I sought did exist. Wendy's grave. I knew I had to see it, but I wasn't sure why. I knew other people left stuffed animals, pictures, or flowers on graves. I didn't feel an urge to leave anything. I just wanted to know whether the sun shone on her grave, whether it was nicely tended and whether the little stone bore her name. Did it say "Wendy Carol Lipman, Dec. 18, 1970—Jan. 2, 1971"?

I felt a strong need to go to the one place on earth where her name appears, introduce myself and apologize for not visiting sooner. I felt I owed that to her because in some way, I'm living the life she never had a chance to live. I believe she knows that and helps and protects me, sort of like a guardian angel.

I often wondered if Wendy was checking up on me when she appeared in my recurring childhood dream. For many years, I tried to wring meaning from that dream, especially because I'd had it so many times. My first thought was that it had something to do with being lost in the mall—but if that was the case, and this nice girl was offering to help, wouldn't I have accepted? As I grew older, I thought maybe she was the girl I'd marry, but I didn't feel love-struck when I saw her, just comfortable. She seemed familiar and friendly.

I continued to wonder, if the helpful girl was Wendy, why we met in the mall, and why under a clothes rack? I kept turning it over in my head until I realized I was hiding from something in a big public place and looking for a haven where I felt secure. Maybe the mall was the world and the clothes rack was my own personal haven. The fact the girl found me so easily and didn't seem at all surprised to see me made me think she knew me pretty well and didn't feel she was intruding.

Doing my best Sigmund Freud, I decided that the rack represented cystic fibrosis. I was hiding under it, afraid to venture out and explore the world or try anything new. I was afraid of emerging from the "protection" of my ignorance about CF. Knowing too much might mean I'd have to confront terrifying details, like my life expectancy. Books were pessimistic, and doctors often were, too. But this girl knew I didn't have to go it alone and tried to gently pull me into the world.

I wish I could get back into that dream and at the part where she asks me, "Do you need any help?" instead of saying, "No," I'd say, "Tell me who you are," or "How can you help me?" I don't feel I can manipulate the dream, though I'm curious. I'm not even certain the girl was Wendy, but it's my dream, so its meaning is up to me. I choose to believe the inquisitive girl who appears during times of stress is my older sister, who probably would feel very much at home in a mall. She's just making a guest appearance in my subconscious to check up on her baby bro.

I decided it was time to return the favor and check up on her. In March 1999, nearly three decades after she died, I visited her grave. I wouldn't have been able to do it if I had not thought of an unobtrusive way to get my mom to tell me where she was buried. I didn't want to come right out and ask because I knew Mom would be concerned I suddenly wanted to know and think there was something wrong with me. We talked about Wendy briefly that day over the phone. Mom mentioned how beautiful she was, how much she missed her and how sad it was to lose her. While brief, it was an emotional conversation. I figured now was a good time to get what I needed. I managed to slip the information from her exactly the same way that, when I was a teenager, I'd talk my dad into handing me a few extra dollars for a trip to the baseball card store. I told her I was doing research for a book I planned to write and wanted to be sure I mentioned where my sister was buried.

"Crest Lawn," Mom revealed.

Finding out where Wendy was put to rest was the easy part. Deciding what to do once I was at the cemetery was more difficult. The Jewish custom when visiting a grave is to place a small stone on it to show you've been there. Because this would be my first visit and there was a lot to catch up on, I decided to write Wendy a letter telling her everything I wanted her to know.

I tucked the letter in my pocket and headed to the cemetery on a sunny Saturday morning. I assumed I'd be drawn to her grave, sister tugging brother to the spot. But once I got to the cemetery, there were so many gravestones that I couldn't find Wendy at all.

It was going to be a long morning.

I wandered around the cemetery for an hour hoping my instinct would lead me to my sister's grave. It didn't, but anyone who's seen me get lost driving around Atlanta shouldn't be too surprised. I had to ask for directions to "Babyland"—which sounds like it should be a store that sells diapers and playpens. Instead, it was a section of the cemetery up a little hill with modest gravestones reminding anyone who visited that some of the dead barely had a chance to live.

I took a deep breath of chilly spring air and began to look for my sister. Holmes ... Shields ... Lipman. Wendy Carol Lipman. Nothing more, but that was enough. I'd never seen the stone before, yet I knew when I saw it that it was something I'd been searching for my whole life, even before I knew it existed. I looked at the cropped grass on the plot in front of the marker and sunk to my knees to get as close as possible to her. I felt a little queasy. I took a deep breath and looked around—there was no one in sight—and read her my letter:

Dear Wendy:

I know you know who I am. I just wanted to thank you for always looking after me. I guess because you check up on me so often, you probably want to know more about me.

I am twenty-five years old. I have dirty blond hair and blue eyes. I'm a spitting image of our father. I inherited his sense of humor as well. Speaking of Dad, I work as a purchasing manager in his company. You'd be really proud of him. The company is doing extremely well.

I went to college at the University of Georgia. I play all sports, including basketball, football, softball and tennis. I work out a lot, and I am writing a book about cystic fibrosis. I assume you know that I have CF, too, but I have been more fortunate than you in that I have been able to overcome much of it. Do I have you to thank? I bet I do.

Wendy, I won't let CF defeat me. My mission for the book I'm writing is to combat CF and tell other people it can be done. I'm sorry you died, but I am happy you will always be with me.

When I ask Mom about you, she talks about how pretty you were and how she misses you. She brings a stuffed animal and flowers to your grave every year on your birthday. I didn't know that you died from CF. Mom told me only because I asked her since I was writing this book. I was shocked. Mom had a difficult time dealing with your death, but she will always love you.

Sometimes I ask myself, "Why did Wendy die, and why did I survive?" Now it doesn't matter because we are in this battle together. We can take care of your murderer. Let me do the writing, and you just help me with what to say. I realized several weeks ago that you were the one in my dream. I want to thank you for always offering me your sisterly advice. I know I have always refused your help because I claim to be fine without it. The truth is, I do need it.

I have so many questions, not only about CF but also about you. Do you watch over me? Was it your idea that I would wake up on my twenty-fifth birthday thinking I should write a book? Do I have CF because God thought I might be able to help myself and others beat it? What's heaven like? Do you hang out with our family and with Howard? If you do, please give him a hug from me, tell him I love him and I'll be thinking of him on his birthday.

I guess you're wondering why I'm here. Well, I'm not sure myself. I guess I just wanted to know that you lived. I feel like part of me is missing because I never met you. Mom and Dad still love you very much. Oh yeah, I have another sister, Emily, who doesn't have CF and is a great kid. Maybe one day you can tell her who you are.

This is the closest I've ever been to your body, but I believe your soul lives inside me. I love you Wendy, and I'll see you in my dreams.

Love,
Your brother Andy
P.S. CF's days of dominance are numbered.

When I finished, the cemetery was silent, except for the birds and the rustle of branches, which were dotted with buds. I ran my fingers across Wendy's name on her gravestone, and as I did, I noticed a small wildflower next to the marker. It was reaching for the sun as if to prove that she was nurturing something beautiful and wanted to share it with me. It was another gift from my sister, a wish from Wendy that I'd be comforted and see that strength could come from pain.

As I walked slowly to the car, I thought all the emotions I felt might overflow and I'd cry. I was surprised when that didn't happen. I realized that the overriding feeling I had was of happiness. Why should I be crying? I'd finally met Wendy.

I felt she'd met me, too, and I felt surer of it after talking to Aunt Susie on the phone one day at work. I told her about the cemetery visit and how comforting, yet disconcerting, the experience was. It made me wrestle again with why anyone should have to die after just sixteen days of life. Susie listened and then told me something she'd never shared before.

"Wendy's death was very hard on your mother," she said. "I've told you she was a broken person after your sister died, but there was an emptiness and longing in her that broke my heart. There was no love or laughter in Eva until you were in her belly. Your survival healed her."

I thought about what my aunt said and it gave me solace. I thought, "It probably makes Wendy happy to know that Mom is content now." I was turning that thought over in my head when a strange thing happened.

One of the temps in the office brought in a fax for me. I figured it was a message from a vendor, so I wasn't in a hurry to read it, but the hand-written note on the bottom caught my eye. It said only, "Thank you, Wendy." I glanced at the top and realized the fax was for someone else at the company. The temp for some reason thought it was mine. For reasons she could never imagine, I knew that though it wasn't addressed to Andy Lipman, the message was meant just for me.

Chapter 24
What Am I About?

Growing up, I did not understand that the way I handled CF would determine how strong I would become. I always wondered how I would cope if I developed a really bad lung infection. I knew that having cystic fibrosis meant a bad infection would occur sooner or later. I'd had one in school, but it was caused by my own apathy. Just weeks after my 26th birthday, while playing softball, I was four-for-four that night, including a home run. My teammates patted me on the back each time I circled the bases and raced to the dugout. While everyone was thrilled at our soon-to-be victory, I sat on the end of the bench lost in worried thought.

During the prior inning, a line drive was smashed my way. Instead of diving for it and making the play, I took it on a hop. A ball I would normally catch while smearing my pants with dirt was, on this night, a ball I could only get to on a hop. When I ran, it felt as if I were carrying a 40-pound weight on my chest. I could hardly breathe. I tried to convince myself it was the humidity, but the humidity wasn't real high on this cold September day in Atlanta. I hated playing at anything less than my best. I was the kind of guy who slid into home plate, even if there was no chance I'd be out. I didn't know how to play sports without giving 120 percent.

Steve Davis, my coach and good friend, saw me moping in the dugout.

"You look a step slow tonight," he remarked. "What happened on that fly ball, Pigpen?"

"Pigpen" was one of my nicknames because, like the Peanuts character, I was always getting dirty. If I didn't scrape my knees sliding into home plate, I was at least going to get a few grass stains making a diving catch. Steve knew 90 percent of my teammates wouldn't have dived for that ball; he also knew I would have.

"I don't know. I guess I got a late jump," I mumbled.

I knew what happened, though. I just didn't want to tell him, my teammates and especially not myself. It wasn't the humidity. It wasn't the fact that I got a late break on the ball. The reason I couldn't catch up to that ball was that a familiar villain had reared its ugly head. Cystic fibrosis, a disease I'd recently taken for granted, was back with a vengeance.

I was sick. After consulting with my parents and a few friends, I knew I had to see a doctor. That night I found every good luck charm I owned, rubbed them and tried to maintain a positive attitude. The following morning I drove to my doctor's office. I figured my lung function numbers were going to be down. The question was how much. They were usually in the 95 to 100 percentile, which was excellent for a CF patient. These numbers reflected how much air I could breathe in and how much I let out. I thought maybe my stats would be 10 percent below the usual, 15 at the absolute maximum. That was my worst-case scenario. I was floored when the doctor told me my numbers had plummeted to the low seventies, a decrease of nearly 30 percent. Doctors were concerned when my numbers went down 10. I could see the warning light flashing on my doctor's forehead.

"What do you think it is?" I asked. I wasn't sure I wanted to know.

"Well, it could be pseudomonas."

There was that word again. Pseudomonas was the same bacteria that Dr. Boat worried I had back in my suicidal college days. Once pseudomonas enters the lungs, it gradually destroys lung function until breathing becomes nearly impossible. I had the gall to ask if I could play softball the next week. He recommended I take the rest of the year off to get better. Then he showed me my test results and reeled off all the medications needed to keep my health from getting worse. Not to get better, just not to get worse!

It didn't help that my regular doctor was out of town. He was a very positive man and could usually motivate me to think positively, too. He'd tell me I was stronger than he was, a true compliment from a doctor to a cystic fibrosis patient. He'd always confer with Dr. Boat before making any changes in my routine. This doctor didn't know me and just laid out the facts. I didn't want facts, though. I wanted the silver lining. Like every patient, I wanted the good news.

I had a lump in my throat and an awful feeling that I was in a war I wasn't sure I could win. That wasn't like me. At least, lately, I hadn't been like that. I was a tough guy. I'd battled CF before, but this new infection was the worst I'd faced. It wasn't like the one in college where I could start doing my therapy, taking meds and exercising and I would be on the road to recovery. I was already doing these things. I was giving 100 percent of myself, yet my health was still failing. That was the scariest part.

I dialed my mom as soon as I got in the car. "My numbers are down. The doctor said it could be pseudomonas," I told her. I tried to take a deep breath, but I couldn't hold back my tears.

"Andy, it's okay. It's not pseudomonas," my mom said.

"What if it is?" I cried. "I don't want to die, Mom. It's beating me."

"It's not," she insisted, trying to hold back her own tears. She refused to consider otherwise, which scared me as well. She didn't know any more than I did.

During the next few weeks, things didn't get much better. I lost fifteen pounds. With cystic fibrosis, weight loss is a sure sign that the patient's health is deteriorating. Most CF patients don't like to lose weight, not even a few pounds. We don't go on diets except to gain weight. People with cystic fibrosis need the extra calories because it's tougher to absorb the nutrients and fats in foods. The more calories consumed, the better prepared the body is to fight infection. My declining weight wasn't the only issue. I couldn't talk without coughing and I'd lost my voice from all the medications I was ingesting.

I thought of the philosophical question: "What am I about?" I acted like I could beat cystic fibrosis, but maybe I couldn't. Was I a hypocrite for telling people that CF was beatable when I was not sure I could beat it myself? What did that kind of negativity say about my attitude? Why was it when anything happened to me, the first thing I thought about was death?

I waited a week for the results of my sputum culture, a week of not sleeping, excessive coughing and ungodly fear. Every time the phone rang, I caught it on one ring. I was afraid to find out what I had, but I had to know so I could understand what I was dealing with. More than anything, I needed a good night's sleep and I couldn't do that without knowing my prognosis. I watched the phone, as if it were an opponent at the poker table. "Come on," I thought. "Ring!"

Finally I got the call from Dr. Cohen, who had just returned from a conference. I could hardly speak. Thankfully, Dr. Cohen did most of the talking. He told me the infection I had was staph and not pseudomonas. While I was relieved, I was not out of the woods. Staph was very serious, but I'd had it before. This infection, however, was by far the strongest I'd ever experienced.

The following day, I e-mailed Steve and told him my season was most likely over. I'd never told him or my teammates that I had cystic fibrosis, and I felt increasingly demoralized with each keystroke. Softball was more than just a game to me. It was normalcy. It was six innings of not having to think about cystic fibrosis. Steve e-mailed back that when I was better, he would insert my name right back at the top of the lineup.

As the doctor advised, I took it easy for the next few weeks. Fortunately, I was working with my father, who understood how essential it was that I take an extended sick leave. I became familiar with the mid-morning talk shows. I hated doing nothing, but I was reminded with each breath how important it was to rest. I felt as if I had a large tissue lodged in my throat that wouldn't let me breathe comfortably.

I was pretty depressed the first few weeks. Cystic fibrosis had come out of hibernation like a bloodthirsty vampire and attacked when I least expected it, but after a month or so my pulmonary numbers were a little better. I went to the doctor every week, and was taking more meds than I'd ever taken in my life. I was exhausted, but I was able to start working half days, leaving the office at two o'clock to rest and get my health back. My energy level was still extremely low.

I was being as cautious as I could, trying to follow the doctor's orders. I realized that the doctors were probably right. Running around on a dirty softball field was probably not a good idea for someone so sick, especially on cold autumn nights. Maybe taking the rest of the year off was the right move.

As my first full day back at work ended, I was checking the plethora of e-mails I'd amassed from earlier in the week. Sitting there, I could only think about one thing. On the other side of town, my softball team was gathering for another game. This would be the fifth consecutive week I'd missed the game. The doctors didn't want me rushing back to play sports and I got the feeling they didn't think I'd be able to play again. The question came to me once more: What was I about? Was I someone who was tough only when things weren't so bad, or was I someone who could step it up when things got difficult?

That afternoon, I sent my friends with CF an e-mail saying I was considering playing that night . . . against doctor's orders. My cleats, jersey, bats and glove were stowed in the back of my beat-up black Ford Explorer. Our game started in less than an hour. I told them I wanted to play and that I badly wanted to beat cystic fibrosis. The e-mail was very powerful and uplifting, but it hid the fact that I was afraid to go out on that field and risk my health.

A brief coughing spasm ensued, as if to remind me about the crippling effects of cystic fibrosis. As someone who dealt with the disease for more than a quarter century, I didn't need the reminder.

Some people in my situation might ask for a miracle. I realized a long time ago that hoping for miracles wasn't going to change anything. If anything was going to change, I had to make it happen. I had to go back to working hard in the gym, taking the proper meds and, at the same time, being careful not to overdo it.

I finally made the decision to hold off playing. I would take extra special care of myself and make my first priority my health. I'd always been a competitive person, but now perhaps I needed to slow down and accept that cystic fibrosis was a deadly disease. It could beat me. Though I'd had rough times, I'd lived a higher quality of life than most people ever expected.

As I was preparing to shut off my computer and head home, another e-mail popped onto my screen. It was from a young girl named Connie who had CF, but her battle had been much more difficult than mine. She'd read my e-mail about possibly playing that night. She and I had e-mailed very little in the past, but I knew she, like most of us with cystic fibrosis, needed faith in something or someone.

"Andy, I love the attitude. Hit a homer for me!!!" Connie cheered.

How could I disappoint a young girl who needed to believe in someone? I returned her e-mail and promised that I would hit a homer for her. In fact, I e-mailed all of my friends with cystic fibrosis and promised them that I would circle the bases for them. Anything was possible if I worked hard. I still wasn't 100 percent, but I was sick of lying around hoping I'd get better. I was sick of accepting mediocrity. It was time to take the bull by the horns.

Doctors are well intentioned, and I will listen to them regarding what meds I should take and treatments I should try, but when it comes to being Andy Lipman, that's my job and I take it seriously. Ultimately, I'm the one who knows what I'm about.

After sending the e-mail, I rushed to my car, turned up the Superman soundtrack and drove to the Brookhaven Boys and Girls Club. I had several coughing spasms during the drive, but they did not deter me. I hurriedly put on my uniform and slung my glove and bat over my shoulder. As I stepped onto the worn grass field with its holes and patches from a season full of diving catches, I found Steve putting the final batting order on the lineup card. He welcomed me back with open arms, adjusted the lineup and put me back at leadoff as he promised he would. I got hugs and handshakes from both teams, as I had friends in each dugout.

As I stepped up for my first at-bat, Ira Graiser, my close friend and third base coach, gestured to me that he'd send me home, even if there was going to be a close play.

Prior to the first pitch, another coughing spasm ensued, but I wasn't worried about how crippling CF was anymore. I was thinking more about how amazing it would be to e-mail Connie and tell her that I hit a home run for her. My teammates were chanting "An-dy! An-dy! An-dy!" as I stepped into the batter's box. They knew what I'd been through and were proud of me for getting back on the field.

The pitcher set himself and threw the ball right in my wheelhouse. I clutched the bat, pulled my hips back and hit the ball on a rope toward right centerfield.

"Run," the first base coach screamed, "Run!"

I saw the ball slip by the right centerfielder as he sprinted toward it. As I came around second base, I saw Ira at third base coming through on his promise and waving me home. There was going to be a play at the plate. I was breathing heavily, but still running as hard as I could as I rounded third. The catcher stretched out her mitt for the ball. I looked for home plate and slid.

The following morning, I e-mailed Connie and the rest of my CF friends and told them that while I promised to hit them a home run, I did not hit one. I explained that the most important thing was that I went out there and played as hard as I could. Even when I wasn't sure I could persevere, I still gave it everything I had. For me, and for them, the fact that I beat cystic fibrosis that night was the real home run.

That night still stands out in my mind as one of the most defining moments of my life. That was the night I beat cystic fibrosis. As much as a home run meant to me and to my team, as I grew older that became the less important part of the story. What was most important is that I did not let CF win. I realized no matter how fiercely cystic fibrosis fought me, no matter how much it took out of me, no matter what the doctors said I could not do, I had one thing going for me, and that was drive . . . and I still have that drive at 35!

Oh, and as far as Connie goes, she e-mailed to thank me for inspiring her to work harder. She said it didn't matter if I hit a home run or not. To her, what mattered most was that I went out there and tried.

"All I said was I didn't hit one home run," I e-mailed back. "The operative word was one…. I hit two."

That's what I'm about!

Chapter 25

A Wish Comes True

In the spring of 1999, I was at an event called the Cigna Sports Challenge, which benefited the Cystic Fibrosis Foundation. They raised money by doing all sorts of small games like miniature golf and tug-a-war. A buddy from my softball team was running the event and asked his teammates to volunteer. I decided to help, but told no one there I had cystic fibrosis.

It was a beautiful day in Atlanta. I saw smiles on all of the volunteers' faces, as well as the competitors. The curious thing was the losers in these games didn't get mad. "It was for a good cause," one said. I'd never actually seen people compete without getting flustered after losing. That's what a great event and cause can do.

The Atlanta Falcons cheerleaders were there, and so were two special people. Two little girls with cystic fibrosis stood up and thanked everyone. I whispered to myself, "I'm like you. Wendy was like you." It was the first time in a long time I'd seen anyone with cystic fibrosis. I realized I'd never done anything for people like me. I thought of Wendy, who never had a chance to live, and how I'd never done anything for the fight against the disease we shared. No one even knew I'd had an older sister. It was as if she never even existed. But I knew that she did. I wanted to do something meaningful in her memory. It was then that a light bulb went off in my head.

I wasn't enthusiastic about tug-of-war or any of those games. The game I loved was softball. I wanted to combine my love of softball with my passion to beat cystic fibrosis and honor my sister's memory at the same time. I would add a few ideas I got from the Cigna Sports Challenge to a few of my own.

The idea gained steam one night at my friend Shira's house. We'd talked about how cool it would be to have a little softball tournament with all of our friends. Shira, who helped organize a lot of fundraising events, enthusiastically suggested that we could do it for charity. That thought was already foremost in my mind. We'd do it to benefit those with cystic fibrosis and we'd do it to remember my sister. My buddy Seth was included in our three-person planning committee.

A Wish for Wendy Softball Challenge started as a promise to my sister—a promise that she would be remembered and a disease would be destroyed. The proceeds from the event would benefit the Cystic Fibrosis Foundation. I had no idea how to run an event, but one member of my family provided great assistance.

In the late seventies, my mother ran a charity toy donation event called The Santa Claus House. My mom, along with other great volunteers, raised around ten thousand dollars annually for the Cystic Fibrosis Foundation. The Santa Claus House was my mother's first attempt at using her amazing people skills to pull off the seemingly impossible. She'd heard that singer/songwriter Isaac Hayes ran along a certain road in the Buckhead area of Atlanta, most mornings, so the Friday of the event my mother drove that street and lo and behold, she found Mr. Hayes and stopped him in mid-run. Fully aware he might say "no" or just keep running, she made the attempt, anyway. He was very nice and said he'd send some autographed memorabilia. My mom was grateful for his courtesy and thought even if nothing came of it, maybe she raised another person's awareness about this horrible disease.

The day of the event, one of the volunteers approached my mom and said, "There are two big guys here who want to speak to you."

Two broad-shouldered men approached and said they were Mr. Hayes's bodyguards and they had a box full of autographed photos and albums by Isaac Hayes. My mom proved the old adage, "Nothing ventured, nothing gained," and she proved it again at A Wish for Wendy. Since the beginning, mom has been in charge of all the food and has solicited most of our silent auction memorabilia.

Even though I walked into the Cystic Fibrosis Foundation in a nice gray suit, I'm not sure they took me seriously. Maureen Fraser, the head of the chapter, knew my family because they'd done so much for CF awareness in the past. My dad was a member of the board for many years and my mom, of course, ran The Santa Claus House.

I proposed the idea of starting a sixteen-team, single-elimination softball fund-raiser, and Maureen followed by asking me several questions. "How many people do you think will attend? Will this be a one or two-day event? How do you plan to raise money outside of team entry fees? How much will the team fees be?" I didn't have a lot of answers and I wasn't sure I could pull off my grand scheme, but I knew I had to try. I owed it to Wendy.

The first year was a bit of a mess. One team didn't show up. One team didn't have enough players. Two teams got into a verbal war because one of them unknowingly changed their lineup illegally. Half of the players didn't get food because homeless people, who lived at the park, took a majority of our refreshments. The championship game had a controversial call, and the worst thing was that we'd decided because Piedmont Park lacked lighting, tie games would not go into extra innings to avoid playing in the dark. Instead, tied teams would have a home run challenge to decide the winner. Each team picked one person and that guy got one chance to hit the ball; the longest ball would win. As luck would have it, there were no ties until the championship game. Each guy hit one ball, and the championship was won by two feet.

I considered giving up on the event after that, but then someone uttered the words that, since then, I've heard every year, "Andy, we can't wait for next year!"

I got so many compliments from so many people about that event that I decided we would do it again and just make improvements.

Each year the event grew and seven years later, it was a double elimination tournament on four fields with thirty sponsors. A Wish for Wendy went from raising thirty thousand dollars annually for cystic fibrosis research to one hundred twenty thousand. It went from being a little known gathering of friends at a park to having far reaching public appeal.

We also started an annual silent auction that raises thousands of dollars, thanks to many generous donors who contribute sports merchandise and other items. In the last few years A Wish for Wendy attracted teams from all over the state of Georgia, as well as dozens of wonderful volunteers. Despite the changes, many of the same teams come out every year to compete. People travel from as far as Illinois, Rhode Island and Mississippi to be in Atlanta on the first Saturday in November to compete on the softball diamond. Every year the success of A Wish for Wendy reminds me how fortunate I am to have the amazing friends and family that I have.

Traditionally, we've had a celebrity draft for teams that raised the most money. These celebrities included All-Star Brian McCann from the Atlanta Braves, Emmanuel Lewis from the hit TV series *Webster* and Mike Devereaux, MVP of the 1995 National League Championship Series. We have had some pretty great guests, too . . . the Chick Fil-A cow, the Atlanta Falcons cheerleaders, and several Major League Baseball players, including future Hall of Famer Chipper Jones. We've also received support from the Garth Brooks Teammates for Kids Alliance.

In its first twelve years, A Wish for Wendy raised more than a million dollars for the Cystic Fibrosis Foundation, whose mission is to find a cure for this deadly disease. The day of the tournament honors my sister's memory, but on that day Wendy isn't just part of my family, she's part of every family that supports cystic fibrosis research. I always feel that I'm living my life for both Wendy and myself. I know if she were here, that she would be living hers to the fullest.

In 2007, we established the Wish for Wendy Foundation to help raise awareness of cystic fibrosis. As part of the effort, I make speeches to civic clubs and professional organizations, at radio stations and schools. The proceeds from these and other events the foundation coordinates are donated to the Cystic Fibrosis Foundation.

I believe that Wendy's wish is for us to find better treatments, so more kids get to live as normally as possible. Selfishly, I wish Wendy could have gotten that same chance, but the important thing is that she will be remembered.

Chapter 26
Who Was That Girl?

For many years, I thought about the girl from the TV movie that my parents prohibited me to watch. Who was she? How long did she live? Was it a true story? These questions plagued me for years.

It took me more than thirteen years to learn the girl's identity and what happened to her. One day I found a website that mentioned Frank Deford, a *Sports Illustrated* writer. His name was familiar to me because I remembered my mom telling me he was involved in the Cystic Fibrosis Foundation and had lost a daughter to CF. I double-clicked on his name and read his biography. It mentioned a book he'd written, *Alex: The Life of a Child*, which had been made into a movie. Aha.

Looking back, my mom did the right thing in not letting me watch the movie. My parents tried to shelter me as much as possible from the negative aspects of CF, so that I could enjoy my childhood without fearing for my life and obsessing about my health. I remembered Mom telling me to ignore the kids in elementary school who taunted me about dying. I also remembered how she refused to enroll me in cystic fibrosis camp because she didn't want me to be around kids who were sicker than I was, and who might get me focused on illness and dying. I knew she didn't tell me how Wendy died because she wanted to protect me from the fears of CF.

Still, I think I would have been better off if I'd known a little more about my disease. As a kid, I didn't know anyone else who had cystic fibrosis. Those friendships were absent from my childhood and teen years, so there was no one I could talk to about it. I could have talked to my parents or my doctors, but that was different. None of them knew what it was like to have CF, and they each had what I thought of as an agenda. My parents tried to be optimistic, whereas the doctors were pessimistic, especially when they talked about the long term.

Though I'd never met Frank Deford, or read the book he'd written about his daughter, I had a hunch he would understand many of my feelings. I sent him a note telling him how much I appreciated his leadership efforts with CF.

I didn't expect a response. After all, the guy was a famous sportswriter who got a lot of mail and who was always very busy. So I was very surprised several weeks later to find a note from him in the mail.

If he had taken time to write me, the least I could do was read his book. I bought it and kept it unopened for several weeks. I knew it had a sad ending—a beloved daughter dies of CF. I finally cracked the cover on an insanely early flight to Cincinnati with my dad for one of my routine doctor's appointments. I was exhausted, having gotten only a few hours of sleep after a late night softball game. However, once I started reading, I couldn't put Alex's story down because so much of her life mirrored mine.

Like me, she'd thought about death, but was afraid to talk about it with her parents. Like me, she was disappointed and depressed because she couldn't keep up with her friends in gym class. She, too, loved her friends because they didn't treat her any differently because she had a life-threatening disorder. And both of us knew what it was like to have cystic fibrosis.

Alex wasn't expected to live longer than a couple of years, but she proved the doctors wrong. I admired her so much for that, for fighting for her life and never giving up. She lived eight years, and her death, though tragic, had a dramatic impact on the country's awareness of cystic fibrosis. Before Alex's story was told in a movie and book, the Cystic Fibrosis Foundation was raising about fifteen million dollars a year. Afterward, contributions for research leapt to one hundred thirty million. So it is due to Alex, really, and the Defords, that I'm as healthy as I am today. I owe her big time.

One of my goals is to finish what Alex started. I want to change the perception people have about those of us with cystic fibrosis. Yes, it's a deadly disease, but the breakthroughs that routinely occur make a cure for CF closer than ever. I also want people to know not to treat anyone with CF differently. As Frank Deford put it so well, "If you start off saying a child is special because she suffers from a handicap, it is a disservice, because you are robbing her of what she might become on her own."

He's right.

While Frank's book is beautiful and the movie is fraught with emotion, I don't want kids with cystic fibrosis to see that movie and think their fate will be the same as Alex Deford's. Things have changed. There are better medications, more CF specialists and a lot of new research being done.

I never thought I'd consider an eight-year-old girl a hero, but Alex Deford was just that.

Chapter 27
The One

In the years after Stephanie and I broke up, I dated a lot. No one special, but it was good practice in meeting girls and being myself. During those years, I began mentioning CF earlier in my relationships. I wasn't afraid to bring it up even on the first date, though I realize that wasn't always a good idea, either. There's nothing like the revelation about having a fatal disorder to turn a promising evening into a polite handshake and, "Thanks, I had a really nice time. Bye."

As positive as I am about my life and my experiences with cystic fibrosis, other people aren't always as knowledgeable or accepting, and sometimes their ignorance gets in the way. I can't control that. I once had a girl back out of a date with me because previously I'd been so sick that I had to cancel. She knew I had CF, and I had to think she was afraid I already had a foot in the grave. I remembered the girl in college who freaked out when she glimpsed me using my therapy machine. I'd seen the worst in women—in men, too, who didn't understand CF, but thanks to people like Stephanie and Bryna, I knew there were a lot who would understand.

In the summer of 1999, my friend Ira wanted someone to go with him to a party. His ex-girlfriend was there and he didn't want to go by himself. I didn't want to go, but Ira eventually talked me into it.

I was enjoying some of the food when I spotted her on the other side of the courtyard. I was immediately struck by her beautiful smile. She had long brown hair, dark eyes, and tan skin. I felt a spark the first moment I saw her. But I soon found there was a lot more to Andrea Herz than her beauty. She was smart—a master's degree from Emory University and a nimble mind that could win an argument with Johnny Cochran—and (thank you, God) athletic. She played football, softball, ran track, swam and excelled at running through my mind.

As Ira and I were leaving, he thanked me for talking to his ex so they didn't have that awkward moment of conversing with each other that exes always detest. I'd never met his girlfriend and had no idea that Andrea was his ex. I knew he wouldn't care if I went out with her, but I asked anyway, because that's what guys do. He gave me permission, but I was too afraid to ask her. After all, I'd only met her once and she didn't know much about me. I figured since we had several mutual friends, our paths would cross again in the near future.

A few weeks later, Ira called to ask if I'd be willing to talk to Andrea, who was going through a tough time. Ira thought my experiences in battling CF might help Andrea with her problem. "Glad to help," I said, telling myself that of course I was just being a pal and had no ulterior motive whatsoever.

So Andrea and I discussed her problem for a few hours over a really nice lunch at Rio Bravo. It turned out Andrea had recently been diagnosed with thyroid cancer. She was enduring multiple treatments and had just had surgery to remove her thyroid. As if that weren't enough, Andrea had been diagnosed with multiple sclerosis, a debilitating neurological disorder. I couldn't imagine living my whole life without any health issues and then suddenly being struck not just once, but twice, with major health problems.

We talked about each other's issues, as if we were comparing battle scars, and eventually the talk turned to more uplifting subjects like sports and family. Afterward, she said she felt better, I know I did, and before long we were talking every day. It just seemed natural to tell her about my problems with CF. She didn't seem bothered at all. If I had told anyone else I coughed up phlegm all the time, that person would wrinkle her nose and say, "Gross." Andrea, though, asked, "What did the doctor prescribe? Is there a treatment you can do?" It didn't hurt that she knew about cystic fibrosis and other diseases because she worked for the Centers for Disease Control and Prevention.

After just one day of knowing Andrea, I felt comfortable enough with her to lay my life story at her feet, so I let her read the first draft of what would become this book. I figured if she were going to take off, she'd at least be able to do it fast and no one would get hurt. But she stuck around in a big way, and her reaction was like no one else's had ever been. She said, "Don't let cystic fibrosis consume you. It's just a disease. It's not you."

I was smitten, but Andrea didn't want to date me. She was very kind when she explained that she thought I was a really good friend and a great guy, but she was busy dealing with health issues and wasn't looking for a relationship. That was ironic. I always worried that health issues would scare off potential girlfriends and now it was a girl I liked who had the health scare. My friends told me to give up and move on.

It was cystic fibrosis, ironically, that lent a helping hand. CF had taught me never to give up, even when others were sure I wouldn't succeed. If I believed in myself, then I could accomplish what other people thought was unattainable. I learned to never quit on my dreams, and Andrea had become mine. Moreover, I wasn't going to let her go because she was having health issues—that would be hypocritical.

Andrea and I continued to be friends, but it was difficult. One night was especially tough. It was Christmas night and most young single Jews circulated to The Duplex, a place in Atlanta where an annual event called the Matzah Ball was held. I was there with a few of my roommates and some women who came into town for the event. It was a fun night with a few of us dancing in the center of the floor. I showed the moves that made me a hit on the Bar Mitzvah scene and were an embarrassment to many of my family members. Suddenly, the door opened and Andrea appeared. She was as beautiful as ever and her faced glowed with excitement, but it wasn't for me. She was with someone else, and she danced with him most of the night. My roommates tried to get me to leave, but I kept dancing as I watched her. One of our out-of-town guests was dancing with me, but I wasn't dancing with her. I was dancing with Andrea . . . at least in my head. One of my roommates finally got me to leave, but that night I began to realize that my chances of dating Andrea were slim. It was time to move on.

I was having some health issues at the time, and I knew my infatuation was unhealthy because it kept me from focusing on getting better. It was then that I decided to see a therapist. I went to Jewish Family Services and began meeting with a psychologist twice a week.

The experience was great. We talked about my health concerns, my feelings about Andrea and my insatiable hunger for achieving goals. I learned that while achieving milestones was positive, the way my mind worked in reaching them was not. I was always thinking about the next accomplishment, rather than enjoying the one I'd just reached. That was something she wanted me to work on. Talking to a neutral person about Andrea made me feel better, because my roommates were beginning to think I was a stalker and I certainly couldn't talk to Andrea's friends about her. I stopped seeing the therapist after ten weeks. She helped a great deal and I learned to take a different approach in many of the things I did.

A few months later, when Andrea moved to Washington, D.C. for a three-month work assignment, I sensed a change. When I told her about women I was dating, she grew increasingly frustrated with me. I suppose I was calling her less because I didn't want to get too attached. She didn't like the fact that I wasn't calling as much and as that summer was ending, I got a call from her. She informed me that she wanted us to date. There were two problems. First off, I did not have a lot of time to talk. I'd bruised tendons in my hand that evening playing softball so I was having a brace fitted for my hand at Northside Hospital. The other problem was she had just returned from being out with some friends and I could tell she'd had a few drinks. I wanted to make sure she was serious so I told her to call back the next morning and tell me her "real" thoughts.

The following morning, Andrea called bright and early to confirm that her feelings for me had changed. She no longer wanted to just be friends. She wanted a romantic relationship. A week later, I welcomed her home to Atlanta. Our first date was August 12, 2000, at a Braves game against the Dodgers. I still have the ticket. My sister and the friend whose place Andrea and I met for the first time, Shira, also attended. Our relationship officially began.

We'd been together for a few months when, one night on the way home from a trip to Knoxville where I'd met her dad for the first time, we plunged into the infamous CF discussion. I knew it so well I could have prompted Andrea on her lines. It went something like this:

"Andy, I've been thinking about the fact that you have cystic fibrosis and probably can't have kids. It's scary," she said. (Cue mournful violin music.) "I've been thinking about it for a long time."

I knew where this was headed. I'm standing at the Greyhound station with a suitcase and a one-way ticket to a dot on the map called Breakup City. But Andrea surprised me. She squeezed my hand, grinned and said, "I'm comfortable with things. I'm cool with adopting. Whatever happens, I'm happy just being with you."

Whoa. Say what? "So you're saying. . . ." I couldn't even finish the sentence.

"Andy, isn't it obvious? I love you," she said. (Chirping birds and soaring orchestra)

Man, oh man! I knew I loved her, but I was worried that maybe she didn't feel the same way about me. The fact that she did was unbelievable, amazing, wonderful and heavenly all at the same time.

Andrea just kept on stunning me. She loves to travel. I mean really travel, not just go to Savannah for a weekend or visit Disneyland. She likes to explore the world. She knew I had to use my chest therapy machine, which, though portable, isn't exactly something I could stuff in a backpack while hiking the Scottish moors. So she was thrilled to learn that I didn't have to lug it with me—as long as someone could administer my therapy. Right then and there, she volunteered to learn how to do it. My mom helped teach her. Talk about a unique bonding experience.

I couldn't have been more in love with Andrea and I realized we wouldn't have been dating at all if I hadn't adjusted my attitude about cystic fibrosis. I'd finally developed a mindset that I lacked with Bryna and Stephanie. I'd thought I'd be lucky to find anyone to date because, after all, I was going to die young and was probably unable to have children. My prospects seemed as low as my self-esteem.

My attitude turned around and I give a lot of the credit to spending time with a therapist. Through those sessions I realized that any girl should feel lucky to have me, and I've got a right to be picky, too. That's not arrogance—it's self-assurance.

For a long time, I blamed my relationship problems on CF, but I've learned to see it differently. Once I found someone who could live with me and my CF, I knew I'd found someone truly special. I'd also learned that it was important to be honest about CF. Not just that I have it and I'll always have it, but that it's part of who I am.

After dating Andrea for nearly a year, I asked her parents for permission to marry her. Surprisingly, both agreed. I thought there would be concerns that their daughter was marrying someone with a life-threatening disease. Plus, I couldn't guarantee them grandchildren.

"My brother had a wonderful marriage that lasted about five years before he died," Andrea's father said. "His wife knew of his condition and it did not deter her from marrying him. From that experience, I learned that you take your joy in life when and where it comes. I have been blessed to have my daughter find such a fine person."

Andrea's mother said, "Even if you have only five years, if they are wonderful, that could be worth a lifetime. No one promises us forever, anyway."

Andrea and I were engaged a month later. I proposed during a game of pool, hiding the ring in the corner pocket of a billiard table. Some might think this too informal, but for Andrea and me it was perfect. It was at the pool table that we had some of our best discussions.

A year later, we were married in a beautiful wedding with 250 guests. My groomsmen were all fraternity brothers, plus my new brother-in-law. I guess my dad was right. These guys did become my friends for life.

Ironically, one of our ketubah signers was Ira. The ketubah is the Jewish contract of marriage, which is signed by the bride and groom, the rabbi, and two witnesses before the wedding. Being a signer is a big honor, and Ira deserved it. If it hadn't been for him, I may never have met my wife.

While Ira's role was key, meeting Andrea would have been irrelevant without my newfound confidence that I had a right to be with someone. I was slowly realizing that there was a wonderful future in front of me and marriage was only the beginning.

A year after we were married, that wonderful future continued as Andrea gathered sixty of my closest friends and family members at Turner Field for my thirtieth birthday. She knew what a big accomplishment it was for someone with cystic fibrosis to turn thirty. The party was the best birthday present I could have gotten. I was surprised by the big thirtieth birthday celebration, but I'd like to think the doctors who diagnosed me early on were even more surprised that I had a thirtieth birthday.

Chapter 28
The Ultimate Honor

During a quiet March day in 2001, I was at work sifting through some orders. An e-mail popped on the screen from my friend, Karl Kandell, Jr.

" . . . Karl has nominated you to help carry the Olympic Flame in the 2002 Olympic Torch Relay, presented by Coca-Cola and Chevrolet. Did you know the passing of the Olympic Flame dates back to the first Olympic Games held in ancient Greece? Now you have a chance to be a part of that tradition by participating in this exciting event."

I never knew how the nomination process worked, but I thought it was a nice that a friend nominated me. I continued to look through orders when another e-mail popped up, this time from my friend, Justine Cohen. It was the same e-mail except Justine's name replaced Karl's. Before I knew it, there were thirty e-mails from different friends, each nominating me for the Olympic Torch Relay. I called Andrea to tell her the amazing coincidence that all those people nominated me.

She said, "Darn, it was supposed to be a surprise. I asked some of our friends to nominate you." I thought that was cool, but I never expected to get the call that I'd actually been selected.

As months went by, I continued to get nominations. I later found out that it didn't matter how many nominations anyone got. What mattered were the nominations that the committee read. In other words, it was quality over quantity and each candidate was evaluated based on their life challenges, community service and other good works. I did not expect to hear from the committee, since I was sure lots of people got nominated. Then toward the end of November, I got an e-mail from Coke, the main sponsor of the torch relay: "Congratulations on being selected as an Olympic Torchbearer in the Salt Lake 2002 Olympic Torch Relay."

I was in shock. I couldn't believe that of the thousands of nominees, all of whom had done amazing, inspiring things, I'd been chosen to receive this honor. I called Andrea to thank her and then e-mailed all my friends to let them know how grateful I was that they thought so much of me.

A few weeks later, I received a letter and my uniform. I was to run with the Olympic Torch in Athens, Georgia on December 4, 2001. I donned the Olympic jumpsuit and Andrea and I drove to Athens where we met my cousin, Jonathan, his future wife Laura, my mom and dad, Emily, Aunt Susie and her family, and Nana Rose. Josh and Marci (a close friend of Andrea's) were also there.

Arriving at the Olympic bus stop in Athens, Georgia was like going back to college orientation. I spent several hours getting to know a group of people, but instead of spending the next four years with them, it would only be about four hours.

We were all from different parts of the state. Each person on the bus had a personal story to tell. One was a cancer survivor. One man built houses for Habitat for Humanity. Each was an impressive individual. The only thing we had in common was our excitement about running a two-tenths mile stretch with the torch.

Waiting to run with the torch was like nothing I'd ever experienced. At the pick-up location, we lined up by our torchbearer number and sat in that same order on the bus. We stopped at the top of the hill at a gas station where I'd done some shopping during my undergraduate days and I became a make-shift tour guide for those who had never been to the University of Georgia. After a thirty-minute wait, the bus proceeded to the first stop.

We were called off the bus one-by-one to wait for the flame to be passed to our torch. We each had our own torch, which we were allowed to keep. Finally, it was my turn to walk through the aisle and skip down the stairs. When the bus left, I stood there, torch in hand, waiting for the flame to come my way. The sky was pitch black. I could hardly see a thing. Then, suddenly, a small light came into view. As the seconds passed, it grew brighter and the crowd around me grew louder. The woman, a cancer survivor I'd met earlier, tilted her torch down and I aimed mine towards hers. Voila, the flame was passed. A truck a few feet in front of me began to move. The guy in back focused his camera on me as I ran.

Holding the torch high, I thought how fitting it was that my run happened to take place in Athens. This was the place where I'd given up on myself and where I conceded that CF had defeated me. This was also the place where my comeback began. It was here that I'd learned to lift weights, to run again, and where I'd discovered that my life did have meaning.

As I ran, just yards away from my fraternity house, I thought about Brett, and what he had said to me. He was right. I'd made a mockery of my life then, but no more. I talked to Brett a while ago. He didn't remember our confrontation, but apologized if he hurt my feelings. I told him I should be thanking him for changing my life. Well, I changed my life, but I had him to thank for igniting the flame.

And speaking of flame, my torch lit the streets as I ran. At least that's how it felt to me. I could feel the heat exuding from it as I sprinted down the stretch. Yes, sprinted. Most people jogged, but not me. I wanted to show the world that a person with cystic fibrosis didn't just run with the Olympic Torch, he sprinted the entire way. I burst with pride when I passed my family and friends. I wondered what they were thinking.

Nana Rose had been through the Holocaust. Only in her wildest dreams could she have imagined that her Jewish grandson would run with the Olympic Torch. What were my parents thinking? Twenty-eight years earlier they were told their son would probably die in childhood. They were told he wouldn't do much running because of his lung capacity and here I was sprinting up a steep hill. What must Andrea be thinking? Her one e-mail to our friends had led to this. Then there was Josh. He had always been my chief competitor and here he was rooting for me.

I enjoyed the great Georgia crowds, which are usually only seen on game day. The light from the torch illuminated their excitement as one of their own ran. I shouted, "Go Dawgs!" as I came down the home stretch. I'd never started a cheer before and to hear the fans shout "Go Dawgs!" back at me was a thrill. To have Uncle Bobby there was also nice. After all, it was Bobby who taught me how to run at the Peachtree High School track many years ago. I hoped he knew that I would never forget his contributions to my success.

When the run was over, we each got to write in the Olympic Torch journal that was passed around on the return bus trip. Each person put a lasting impression of what running with the torch was like. All I remember writing was the word, "Amazing" about ten times. I could think of no other word to describe it. On the ride home, I realized what I did that day was remarkably special—something only a small fraction of the population would ever get to do. The number of Lipmans to run with the Olympic Torch would double a few years later when Andrea would also be nominated and would run her two-tenths of a mile in Atlanta. Running with the torch was a tremendous honor but also put a lot more pressure on me. I realized that I was now obligated to do more. While the flame was extinguished from my torch, my efforts to battle cystic fibrosis must never be.

Chapter 29
A New Group of Friends

One of the ironies of having cystic fibrosis is that the people I most wanted to meet—other people with cystic fibrosis—are pretty much off-limits. We each carry hoards of bacteria and, unfortunately, run a big risk of infecting each other with whatever it is that we don't already have. It's really scary because two people with CF can do serious harm to each other without ever intending it, so it's critical that we keep our distance.

That said, I thought it was important to seek out others who have the disease and I found my link to people with CF through the Internet. One day, I landed at the website www.esiason.org, which was created by former All-Pro quarterback Boomer Esiason, whose son, Gunnar, has CF. It has links to medical articles and Esiason's foundation, which were helpful. But what really caught my attention were the profiles of people with CF who were living normal, exciting lives.

One on-line acquaintance, who especially inspired me, was a fellow sports fan named Jason. He played sports, lifted weights and worked for the Charlotte Hornets, a professional basketball team that has since moved to New Orleans. I decided to call him, though I had some doubts about getting in touch. I thought that, like me, he sometimes might not want to talk about CF. Still, I figured I had nothing to lose.

When he answered the phone, I noticed that he sounded great—no gasping for air or wheezing like some with CF. We talked about everything from our infertility to who the Hornets were going to play the next season. Jason was the first person who became not only a friend, but a friend with CF. We e-mailed each other just about every day for a few weeks to share stories, fears and hopes. Over time the e-mails grew farther apart and I eventually lost touch with him. I have since tried to find him, but had no luck. Still, I'd made contact with someone with CF and I realized I wasn't alone. Once I got the taste of a connection, I couldn't stop looking for others who might empathize with me even more.

Before Jason, the only person I'd met with CF was a high school kid who came to examine my therapy machine when I was a teenager. For many years, I thought of someone with CF as someone like him—weak, thin and hoarse from coughing. I also couldn't forget the people with CF I'd seen in doctors' offices. They needed someone to help them cross the room, and many were connected to a network of tubes. The only movie I'd ever seen about CF featured a little girl who died at age eight, and the stuff I'd read about cystic fibrosis said I'd be dead by twenty-five. As much as I disliked the fact that I was stereotyped because of my disease, I was doing the very same thing to others who had it.

Next, I called Kathy, another person featured on the Esiason website. She was an all-star hockey player for Northeastern University in Boston and had been on *Good Morning America* and in *Sports Illustrated*. We talked about how a sense of humor can help keep CF in perspective and how friends' jokes about coughing and other symptoms are actually welcome, because they make us feel accepted. We agreed that it's best for us to ignore news updates about possible cures for CF. We couldn't get too excited about that because we'd been hearing the same thing since we were kids and nothing had happened yet. We needed to be optimistic that one day there will be a cure, but each of us also has to keep taking care of ourselves. Like my relationship with Jason, I have not heard from Kathy in years.

I also found an Internet chat room for CF patients and their families. Soon, I was getting dozens of e-mails each day with questions about everything from medications to insurance. It was a great way to connect with others and share positive energy. Some of the most inspiring messages came from people in their fifties with CF—one was even a sixty-eight year-old man. There are people out there living long lives with CF. That's what I like to hear.

I didn't expect negative stuff, but that was there as well. Some people wrote, "I don't think I can fight it anymore," and even "I wish my parents had never had me." I'd been e-mailing a woman named Letitia, who was going into the hospital for surgery. She wrote back afterward to say she was in pain, but was going to be okay. She died the next day. That really shook me up. I couldn't help but mourn a woman I didn't know, someone who was part of my extended CF family.

It was this aspect of the chat room that disturbed my dad. He thought it attracted people who were needy or negative, not the ones living busy fulfilled lives and just happened to have CF. I know he was afraid negative comments and cold realities like Letitia's death would drag me down, and to some degree, they did. More of my on-line contacts passed away, some I knew very well and others with whom I'd only exchanged e-mails once or twice. E-mails seemed to surface once a week announcing the passing of one of our friends. Death is a part of life, though, and dying at an early age, well, in the cystic fibrosis world, that's reality. For me, however, the benefits of using the chat room far outweighed the negatives.

One of the most important things the CF chat room did was dispel my stereotype of people with cystic fibrosis. Getting in touch with so many who had CF made me realize that we come in all varieties. Sure, some people are sickly, but many, like Jason and Kathy, are healthy, active and optimistic.

I even found my CF kindred spirit on the Cystic-L website. Though I've never met Michelle Smidt in person, we really hit it off. Michelle loves to hike and her goal is to climb down and then back up the Grand Canyon—just to prove that someone with cystic fibrosis can do it. I love that attitude, and I understand it so well. It's the same perspective I have whenever I step up to bat or pause for that split second before making a jump shot. We understand each other perfectly. She's certainly been a huge comfort and help. One of her great lines was, "I have cystic fibrosis, but it will never have me." I never forgot that.

We found that we have much in common. We both work full-time jobs, which is a rarity for adults with cystic fibrosis. Her father has a hard a time dealing with CF, like my mom does. Both feel very protective of us and neither likes to accompany us on doctor's appointments. They love us so much and don't want to see us in any pain. No one else understands the confusions this parental relationship causes better than Michelle.

I dream about meeting Michelle one day. I was invited to her wedding, but quite honestly, I was afraid to go. There is always a risk; I didn't want one of us to give something to the other. I know that sounds weak, but I grew up in a household where staying away from germs wasn't just recommended, it was a mandate. I think we can't be too many years from a test that will detect if people with CF are carrying anything that is dangerously contagious. Once we know we are both okay, Michelle and I will finally get together.

Sometimes the biggest obstacles and disappointments in our lives turn out to be the biggest gifts. I think it's a matter of being grateful for what we have. I went to the Cystic-L site looking for information, but what I found was more than that. I discovered a friend in Michelle. She and I still talk pretty frequently and compare notes in the "fighting CF" department. I hold tight to her friendship because it strengthens me as much as my friendship strengthens her. That's real friendship.

Chapter 30
Slim to None

"You can't win!" That's the famous line Rocky's wife, Adrian, his biggest inspiration in all of the Rocky boxing movies, says to him in *Rocky IV*, when she finds out he is going to fight Ivan Drago, the champion Russian boxer who had just killed Rocky's friend in the ring. I use that same line whenever bad news comes my way. I react to it as Rocky did—with defiant determination. I repeated it and repeated it after I got this e-mail ten years ago:

"Andy, I got it today. I wasn't sure if they contacted you directly . . . but it appears not. I'm afraid the results found a suboptimal sample of sperm in the specimen, suggesting if that sample is an average one for you, it would not result in a conception. I am heading to Florida early tomorrow. Otherwise, I would have preferred to have told you this in person, or over the phone. Stay well, and I'll be in the office all next week if we need to talk."

That was the e-mail from Dr. Cohen that turned my life upside down. I knew the odds of a male with cystic fibrosis conceiving a child were minimal at best, but when it came to cystic fibrosis, I was usually able to beat the odds. I was single at the time, but I wanted to find someone and settle down. I thought it was only fair to know these results so I could be upfront with anyone I dated seriously. I thought maybe I'd be one of the few unaffected by cystic fibrosis in this aspect and be able to have children the same way most people did. If cystic fibrosis has taught me anything, it's that it's never going to be easy. I was twenty-five years old and I was being told that these odds were insurmountable. I was not going to be a father.

I thought back to my childhood and remembered how my dad brought me a souvenir T-shirt and cap from his business trips. I remembered the smell of cotton candy the first time my dad and I went to a Braves game. I remembered when my parents took me to the circus. Now I was being told I'd never have the chance to do these things with my own children.

This devastated me, and I found it hard to talk to anyone about it. Because none of my friends had kids yet, I didn't think they'd understand and I didn't want my parents to feel worse that CF—the disease I inherited from them—had put another roadblock in my way. Besides, I didn't even have a girlfriend at the time, so it seemed silly to make a big deal about it. I wanted to leave work early that day, but I told myself that this would not get me down. I'd been through worse. I decided to turn the negativity of Dr. Cohen's e-mail into my motivation to one day do whatever it took to have a child.

Being infertile wasn't really something to tell a girl on the first date. "Hey, Tiffany, I had a wonderful time. Maybe we could do this again. Hey, and if you're worried about taking the pill, don't be. I'm as sterile as an alcohol wipe. So, can we say next Friday?"

Fortunately I met someone who was able to deal with the fact that having a child would be a real challenge; Andrea recognized that we were meant to be together, whether or not we ever had children.

Still, I couldn't get over being told I couldn't have kids. I was used to statistics and tests telling me the odds were slim. I was also used to changing the odds through positive thinking and hard work. I decided I wasn't going to let one e-mail determine whether I would have a family or not. I would face this challenge like any other.

Talking with Andrea about having kids was hard for me. I was sure she had dreams of her own about raising a family, so it was difficult to break it to her, even though, as someone with an extensive amount of medical knowledge both professionally and personally, Andrea wasn't totally unaware of the situation when she began dating me.

Here's how Andrea remembers it: "I looked at it this way. With all of the medical advances these days, the odds can change. I was willing to be a parent any way I could. Being a mother was the most important thing. It didn't matter whether it was IVF, sperm donation or even adoption. I wanted to be a mom, and I wanted Andy to have a chance to be a dad."

Andrea and I discussed the options for having a child that she researched. I had thought about it briefly, but it made me feel selfish. I knew there were procedures Andrea would have to go through to have a child with me, and that the odds of success, while improved, were not favorable. Our only choice to have biological children was to seek assistance from a fertility clinic. If it didn't work, how would we react? Would it affect our marriage? Would it affect our sanity? Would it destroy our happiness? We had to weigh those factors.

Emotional stress was not our only concern. Since I have to stay away from germs, we would have to get a nanny. Daycare would be out of the question. A nanny is more expensive than daycare. Then there's the time issue. I do an hour or two of therapy every day in addition to working nine to ten hours. When would I have time for a baby? What if Andrea needed a break or was out of town? How could I watch a baby and do my therapy at the same time? I'd have a nebulizer in my mouth, a vibrating vest on my chest, and a baby on my lap. It just didn't seem feasible. What if I got sick? Would I have to wear a mask? Could I still take care of the little one?

Andrea and I weren't the healthiest of people. She had survived thyroid cancer and had multiple sclerosis. I was battling a disease with a median life expectancy in the mid-thirties. Would we be able to beat the odds and be good parents? Then there's the logistical issue of my twenty or so bottles of pills. I would have to hide them in a secure place so the baby would not have access to them. There were other concerns about traveling with a baby and carrying everything we'd have to bring. I already had a therapy machine, an aerosol machine, and multiple bottles of pills, so traveling with a baby and all he or she required would be the equivalent of moving day.

Once I got beyond the emotional duress and the health uncertainties, there was the question of finances. Fertility clinics were quite expensive and were not covered by our insurance. The cost could be upward of fifteen thousand dollars per attempt. Talk about pressure! I was also a carrier of the cystic fibrosis gene, which meant my son or daughter would at minimum be a carrier. That didn't concern me as much as the worst-case scenario—our child having cystic fibrosis. Andrea would have to be tested. If she had the gene, there was no use trying. Adoption was probably out because most adoption agencies would not work with people who have our medical conditions.

Then there were the physical aspects of fertility treatments. We'd both endure uncomfortable procedures, but Andrea would have to undergo the brunt of the physical anguish. I'd have a tough time with that scenario. After all, I was the reason we'd have to go through these fertility procedures.

There were so many reasons against having a baby. And there was only one reason in favor: Andrea and I desperately wanted to be parents. We wanted the chance to be a real family, to love and nurture our children into happy, productive adults, and enjoy our grandchildren in our later years. To us, that reason alone was far more important than all the negative reasons combined.

The decision seemed to be made for us one night when we met a couple of our friends for dinner and to play games at Dave & Buster's. Andrea and I came to a machine that morphs two people's faces and shows what their kid would look like. We decided to try it. First, we had a girl. Then we had a boy. To be honest, neither of the kids was that pretty, but still, it got us thinking that it was time to try and have children.

The one good thing about our situation was we didn't have to go through the frustration of trying and then wondering why things weren't working. Before we were married, Andrea knew we'd need assistance to have a baby.

Once our decision was made, our next step was to find a fertility clinic. Andrea and I asked around and the next thing I knew we'd joined a new club.

Chapter 31
The "Other" Club 1150

In the '90s, midtown Atlanta had a popular night spot called Club 1150 where people in their twenties and thirties gathered. I'd been a regular there as a single guy, but seldom went anymore. Now it was time to visit another Club 1150: Building 1150 in North Atlanta, the offices of Reproductive Biology Associates (RBA).

A year after Andrea and I celebrated our thirtieth birthdays, we walked into "Club 1150" for the first time. I knew just by looking at the other patients that no one wanted to be recognized. Hardly anyone said a word, and in some cases I could tell from a couple's body language which of the two was responsible for them being there.

That day, we began working with Dr. Carlene Elsner. I immediately felt comfortable with her when I saw a University of Georgia diploma hanging on the wall. I quickly pointed out to Andrea that there was not a University of Tennessee diploma. We liked to tease each other about our favorite college football teams.

Dr. Elsner liked football, too, and was a big Dawgs fan. She listened to our story, then explained that before we did anything, I would have to see Dr. Michael Witt, a male infertility specialist, who would determine if I had viable sperm. If I didn't, we would have to use a sperm donor or find another way to have a baby.

I mentioned that tests had determined my sperm was sub-optimal. She explained that meant once it came out, it was sub-optimal. It could be viable in the testicles, but unable to reach the penis. So right off the bat, we were going to find out if I could even have a child. If that was successful, Andrea would be tested for all the CF genes. It's not that I wouldn't love our child if he or she had CF, but I wouldn't want my child to face the same challenges that I had to face if I could help it.

A few days later, I saw Dr. Witt, a fit man with a dark mustache and short brown hair. When I walked in, I thought I was in a *Magnum, P.I.* episode because he looked just like Tom Selleck. Pictures of him running marathons covered his walls. Seeing Dr. Witt as an athlete reminded me of running the Peachtree. I took that as a good sign.

Dr. Witt explained what we'd have to do. "First," he said, "we'll have to see if your sperm is at the optimum level. If it's not, we'll insert a needle into your scrotum so that soon after you'll feel no pain and then…."

First, I thought, if someone sticks a needle in my scrotum, I imagine I'll feel some pain. Second, I don't know why, but I thought in this day and age of advanced medicine, they would use a laser or something less invasive.

"… and then we'll pump the semen from your testicles and we can see if we get enough to give us a fighting chance," Dr. Witt concluded.

So, not only would I have to have this done, but we'd have to do a dry run (pardon the expression) to see if this could even work.

But first, we had to verify if the procedure was even necessary. I was shown to a private room with an assortment of adult magazines and videos and a cup to retrieve sperm. I must admit, I felt a flush of embarrassment when I left. I tried to act as if I'd just been browsing in a library, but I was sure everyone in the clinic knew exactly what I was doing.

A few days later, Dr. Witt's office called to confirm my sperm was indeed sub-optimal. They'd have to retrieve the sperm using a needle. Soon I was signing a consent form for the procedure, although certain below-the-belt parts of my body were protesting.

The procedure was called TESA, or testicular sperm aspiration. The sensation when a long, sharp needle penetrates the scrotum is truly one that I cannot explain in words. The words I actually used were "Oh, my God!" but that doesn't really do it justice.

A few days later, the doctor gave us the news that the procedure worked and that Andrea and I could try to have kids. The reason the "strong" sperm could not be ejaculated was that my *vas deferens*, the duct through which sperm travels to the urethra, was non-existent, a common condition for CF patients. This is due to the large amount of mucus that prohibits the duct from developing.

Andrea was given a blood test to determine if she had any of approximately eighty-eight different cystic fibrosis gene variants. This was called a CF Carrier Screen. Thankfully, the results determined that Andrea was not a carrier of the tested variants, and the odds any of our children would have cystic fibrosis were astronomical. There are actually more than a thousand CF gene variants, but most are very rare and not included in the test. Some are probably still unknown.

Andrea had to deal with tenfold more than I did, so I tried not to complain around her. She would have to handle cycle monitoring and give herself an injection in her stomach every day for over a month to stimulate egg production and to control the timing of ovulation. Twenty-one days after her next menstrual cycle started, she began the daily injections. After the second cycle started, she needed to give herself two shots a day until the eggs were harvested. This helped to maximize the number of eggs produced, and therefore the probability that one would be fertilized.

When it comes to IVF, every step is determined weeks ahead of time. There is no saying, "I'll try to come in today, but definitely tomorrow." Everything is done at an exact time for a reason. Six days into her second cycle, Andrea was going to the doctor every day for blood work and vaginal ultrasounds. This was so the doctors could monitor the follicles—which release the eggs that were growing—know how large the eggs were, and when to harvest them.

Before fertilization, Andrea and I went into "Club 1150" yet again and put on gowns and socks. The socks were ours to keep. Wow, I thought. Fifteen-thousand dollar socks! Andrea left for a few moments and returned with IVs hooked up. She would soon be under anesthesia so the eggs could be removed from her uterus.

Next, I was taken to the operating room where Dr. Witt asked me which testicle I wanted to use for the injection. "Neither" was not an option, so I chose the right one, thinking, "I'm right-handed, so what the heck." He gave me a shot of local anesthetic, which caused a sharp pain that only lasted a few seconds, then pulled out a big needle connected to a plastic device that fit in his palm to collect the sperm. He inserted the needle about half an inch into the testicle and removed a small sample of tissue.

An andrologist separates the sperm from other tissue by placing the sample in a special medium. The medium triggers the sperm to break away, which is the first step in capturing it for the fertilization process. Another special fluid is added to slow the sperm, enabling the andrologist to catch them. During the TESA procedure, as many as two hundred thousand sperm may be collected. The process takes roughly thirty minutes.

Dr. Witt let me pick the music in the room while this was going on. I ruled out Pat Benetar's "Hit Me with Your Best Shot," and ended up choosing Elton John, for no reason at all. He was just the first artist who popped in my head. Dr. Witt and I talked about the new *Star Wars* movie, *Desperate Housewives* and how Billy Joel is an excellent live performer. I guess it was supposed to take my mind off things, but with two nurses holding my arms and a needle extracting sperm from my testicle, call me crazy, but I was focused on that. When we finished, the doctor and his nurses left me alone in the room to clean up.

Andrea's procedure took longer. The first cycle they retrieved twelve eggs, which I found out was okay, but not great. We were reminded that not all twelve eggs would be fertilized and not all of those fertilized would be "A" or "B" grade. Some were "C" and "D" grade, which were pretty much useless.

Next, they delivered the sperm and eggs to a Petri dish. We were told to go home and rest for the remainder of the day and then go back to our normal routines. The clinic called every day to let us know how many fertilized and split. Unfortunately, the number dwindled from seven to five and by the time of the implantation date we were down to three. Within seventy-two hours of egg retrieval, the embryos were transferred into Andrea's uterus through a thin tube gently inserted through the cervix. This non-surgical procedure was performed under ultrasound guidance and Andrea did not need to be sedated. We were even given pictures of the embryos afterward, which basically looked like small cells. Though we didn't send them to our parents as holiday cards or anything, they still looked better than the pictures of the kids we morphed at Dave & Buster's.

Prior to the embryo transfer, we discussed how many we wanted to implant and how many we wanted to freeze. We had five minutes to decide. They should have played the *Jeopardy* theme while we discussed it. In the end, we did not have any to freeze, as there weren't enough of good quality. Still, deciding how many and which ones to implant was tough. We used the expertise of our doctors to make the decision. They chose to use all three embryos. Andrea was told to rest the remainder of the day to maximize the chance that she would get pregnant.

Of course, resting for the remainder of the day was a challenge, since the embryo transfer was the same day as the A Wish for Wendy Softball Challenge. But, that was the one date the doctors felt would give us the best chance at a successful transfer. I'd put two people in charge while Andrea and I drove to RBA, had the implantation, and returned. Other than our family and the two people in charge, no one knew where Andrea and I were going.—and we preferred to keep it that way. I thought it would be wonderful if an event to remember my sister would also have a connection with the birth of our child.

For the next two weeks—and as I had done a few days prior to the transfer—I injected medication into Andrea's hip muscle to improve our odds of having children. I'd only given a shot one time before and that was when I wanted to administer medicine that helped Andrea with her MS. I had to stick it in her thigh. After procrastinating for five minutes, I finally did it, but mentally it drained me so much that I could not do it again. I felt pathetic, but I just couldn't get the nerve up to do it again. First, I didn't want to hurt her. Second, I wanted to do it right.

Attempting the fertility injections wasn't much easier. A fertility injection isn't one of those things that can be done just pretty well. It had to be done perfectly.

After talking to friends who had gone through a similar IVF experience, I finally got up the nerve to stick Andrea in the hip. It was not easy, but each night I was motivated by the pictures of our morphed "kids." We placed the pictures of our morphed children conceived at Dave & Buster's within view while doing the shot for inspiration. Every night between nine and ten we turned on the eighties music channel and put a towel under Andrea to protect the bed from any blood. It was important to do it within the same hour every night. Andrea, or sometimes the doctor, drew two black circles on her hip with a marker. Some people don't require this, but it helped me aim. After I swabbed her with alcohol, stuck in the needle and injected the medication, I massaged her hip area for twenty minutes and concluded by putting a hot compress on the area to relieve the pain and help disperse the medication. These progesterone shots were meant to increase and enrich the blood supply to Andrea's uterus and make it more inviting for the embryo to implant.

Two weeks later, Dr. Elsner called, "Sorry guys," she said, "but you're not pregnant."

Neither Andrea nor I left work early that day. We decided to tough it out because we'd heard that IVF was full of pitfalls and we were determined to stay strong. We stopped the shots. They were meaningless. As much as we hated doing them, we wanted more than anything to do them again—if it meant we were going to have a baby. When the doctors told us to stop everything, it made us feel like everything we'd done was a waste of time.

It was a setback, but Andrea and I decided to try again. We had agreed that we'd try three times. If each of those attempts failed, we'd look at other avenues to have children. Later, we became concerned when Dr. Elsner told us she'd miscalculated, and our chances weren't as good as she originally thought, based on the overall quality of Andrea's eggs. Our doctor didn't give numbers or percentages. She just expressed concerns, and her concern for us was the poor quality of the embryos. That was a downer, but our odds were better than many couples. At least Andrea was producing eggs and, based on her blood levels, the eggs did try to implant.

Dr. Elsner was an awesome doctor. She told us, "We're going to get you pregnant, guys. We're going to get this figured out." We loved her confidence and we got the feeling that if anyone could get us pregnant, she could.

A few months later, we were back at "Club 1150." We saw several friends this time, but there was unspoken promise among us that we wouldn't tell anyone else we'd seen each other there. We were comforted to know we weren't alone, although we wished those couples didn't have to experience the unknown fears or fertility trials.

We repeated the same procedure as last time with a different retrieval protocol to get a better egg quality. This time Andrea produced sixteen eggs. That was promising. The doctors did a genetic test called a PGD-FISH on the embryos to rule out the weaker ones. This test also detected propensity for disorders like Down, Turner's, or Klinefelter's syndrome. This exam also decreased the changes of the embryos implanting.

Again, timing is key to a successful IVF, and it happened that our embryo transfer was on Valentine's Day. I thought that might be an omen. Maybe an event to celebrate our love for each other would help bring Andrea and me the joy of a new baby.

During this attempt, Andrea again noticed some vaginal bleeding. We tried to remain optimistic: some couples had seen blood and still were pregnant. Andrea wanted to take a pregnancy test, though the doctors told her not to because it was too early in the process to be reliable. Despite my pleas, Andrea took the test and the results were negative.

I called the nurse, hoping she would tell us the test didn't prove anything. She said many women experience vaginal bleeding throughout their pregnancy and that a pregnancy test done this early was not going to reveal anything. This was a slight relief, but we had a bad feeling.

Our second IVF attempt seemed to have a black cloud over it from the very beginning. That first day, I was driving home from work when I got a call from Andrea. She was crying and her speech was slurred. I could not understand her. The only word I understood was "died." I thought her dad or mom had died. Finally, I picked up what she was saying and rushed home. Our seven-year old cat, Possum, or as I referred to him, Mr. Possum, was lying on the chair in the guest room, the room we'd decided would be our baby's room. He'd had a heart attack. Possum was the greatest cat and was truly magical. I was allergic to cats, though not to Possum. I was not fond of cats, but loved dogs. So what did Possum do? He acted like a dog. He sat and he fetched. If he had licked, he would have had the trifecta in my eyes. We got him from an old roommate who went into the Peace Corps and couldn't take him. Andrea's only stipulation was that once we took the cat, he was ours. So Possum was our cat and he became our "kid."

That night we covered Possum with the same multi-colored towel we put under Andrea to give the shots and took him to the vet to be cremated. Losing him at that time was not what we needed; we'd been told that trauma makes conceiving even more difficult.

Two weeks later, Andrea called me at the office. "Honey, we're not pregnant," she sighed. She had just gotten the call from Dr. Elsner's office. I could tell that she'd been crying, so this time we both left work early to snuggle and console each other.

Driving home that day, every light that turned red and driver that drove too slowly irked me. I was mad and sad and hurt all at the same time. "Why?" I cried. "Why couldn't I become a father?"

A few months later, Andrea and I tried again. It would most likely be our last attempt. Maybe getting pregnant was not in the cards for us. I wasn't even supposed to live to see my teens, so I shouldn't be disappointed. But we wanted more than anything to be parents.

Chapter 32
A Little Magic in Our Lives

It was the first week of March when Andrea finally succumbed to my begging for a puppy. We needed another body in the house. We'd lost Possum, the greatest cat in the world, and it felt lonely at home. Andrea and I were both big animal lovers. She'd worked as a vet tech for six years and I'd owned more animals than Noah. Andrea never owned a dog. She was more of a cat person.

Andrea and I were determined that we would only save a dog from the pound or a rescue group. In my experience as a dog owner and Andrea's as a vet tech, dogs that were saved turn out to be the sweetest dogs. We went to Atlanta Pet Rescue first. It was a neat establishment with lots of dogs. Volunteers interviewed prospective adopters to determine which dog matched best. We had already checked their website and selected a beautiful husky-shepherd mix named Cinderella. I had called and asked the usual questions of her foster parent. "Does she bark? Is she sweet? Is she house-broken?" The woman answered, "Oh yes, she's a darling. You'll just love her. She's precious."

I was so excited! When we arrived at Atlanta Pet Rescue I had to look through all the smaller dogs to find Cindy. Yeah, I already had her new nickname in my head. I'd even written an e-mail introducing her to our friends to send after we picked her up and got a picture. "Cindy," I jokingly shouted. "Cindy!" Suddenly, a huge dog began barking and growling at the smaller dogs. I gulped. "Cindy?" Andrea tapped me on my shoulder. "That's her all right."

"Cindy," I gasped, "is Cujo!"

Our interview was scheduled for an hour later, so we decided to walk the short distance to the Atlanta Humane Society. We'd pretty much committed to Cinderella and were trying to talk ourselves into getting the little killing machine. "At least, we won't have to worry if the alarm was on the fritz," I thought. "Cindy would scare away the meanest burglars. But gosh, what if she ever got loose?" I was already picturing the news story: "Dog bites kid. Owner goes to jail. News at 11!"

Walking through the pound, we saw a lot of adorable dogs. We could smell that puppy breath wherever we walked. There were many other interesting smells, too, but the cuteness of the puppies kept our focus. Watching the dogs

157

play was pleasant and relaxing. Half an hour later, we realized it was time to leave for our interview. Suddenly, a black twenty-pound Lab/terrier/shepherd mix walked up and began licking my hand.

"She's a licker!" I said with delight.

Andrea turned red and was embarrassed that her husband had a licking fetish, but the truth was I loved affectionate pets.

The dog's name was Tina. She had short black hair and was very cute with the face of a Labrador retriever but the size of a terrier. I'd told myself years ago that I'd never get a black dog because of the Doberman that once bit me, but Tina's eyes made me melt. I could almost hear her begging, "Pick me please." I had already fallen in love with her, but told myself we had to weigh all options, so Andrea and I returned to Atlanta Pet Rescue to give Cinderella a second look.

"Just here to look at Cinderella," I said walking in as if I owned the place. She'd lost her nickname now . . . not a good sign for the four-legged Hannibal Lecter.

We asked when we would be interviewed and the hour-wait was down to five minutes. I looked at all the dogs and then at Cinderella with her piercing eyes and sharp vampire-like fangs. What were we doing here? I didn't want any of these dogs, especially not Cinderella. I had always been the sort of person who did the right thing. It's a curse actually, because sometimes doing the right thing is not what makes you happy. The right thing in this case was wait to be interviewed, since we had signed up and the volunteers were expecting us. I looked at Andrea and she knew what I was thinking. "You think she'll still be there?" she asked.

"We won't know unless we bail." I turned to the interviewer who just called our names and for once, I did the "wrong" thing. "Thanks," I said, "but we're leaving."

We drove to the Atlanta Humane Society, obeying none of the speed limit signs. As I turned into the parking lot, I posed questions in my head. "Maybe Tina licked everyone? Maybe she wouldn't like us the second time? Maybe we didn't give the dogs at Atlanta Pet Rescue a fair shot?"

We walked back to the large play area where Tina and her two siblings were held. People were putting their hands in the pen, but Tina did not move toward them. Fifteen seconds later I knew we'd made the right decision. Tina came right to me and smiled like only a dog can. She licked my hand constantly. Andrea was talking to one of the workers and I looked toward them with Tina's tongue still working away at the salt on my hand. My skin tastes salty because people with cystic fibrosis produce an excessive amount of sweat due to a gland abnormality. I'd known Tina for ten minutes and she was already showing me a benefit of having cystic fibrosis. We had found our dog.

Tina sat in my lap while we filled out the paperwork. It must have been a little strange to see a twenty-pound lapdog. We left her there to get spayed, as that was a rule at the Humane Society.

Less than a week later, I picked up our new dog. She was a little more rambunctious than I remembered, but once I got her in my car, she curled up in the passenger seat and proceeded with her favorite hobby, licking my hand. We decided she should have a new name. We called her Magic. The truth was Andrea and I needed a little magic in our lives, so that's what we called her. I just knew that our little Magic was going to change our lives for the better.

Magic was house-trained in less than a week. Andrea and I'd bought her so many toys our house looked like we already had a child. In a few months she learned to sit, come, turn around, jump, crawl, roll over, and our favorite trick of all, play dead. Andrea taught her that one. It was the trick we showed anyone who walked in the house. A burglar could break into the house and we'd say, "Before you steal everything, watch Magic play dead."

Magic was awesome. She sat next to me every day when I did my therapy. It was as if she knew it was something I didn't like, but that I had to do. It reminded me of Howard and how he sat by me as I watched the other kids play in the yard when I was too sick to go out. Magic would always lie by Andrea when she wasn't feeling well. She loved us unconditionally, and in the same way, we loved her back.

I had to wonder what would have happened if I had done what I usually did and waited for our interview with Atlanta Pet Rescue instead of taking a risk and returning to the Humane Society. I hope Cinderella found a great home, but we needed a little Magic in our lives and that was exactly what we were about to get.

Chapter 33
Third Time's A Charm?

Right after getting Magic, Andrea and I tried for a baby again. During our second trial, everything seemed to go wrong. This time around, things looked better. Andrea's protocol was changed to what was called a flare protocol. Traditionally, flare protocol had a better success rate and this time the doctors were able to harvest twenty-two eggs. That was six more eggs than last time and a remarkable ten more than the first. Some families would be thrilled to have any eggs. It's not automatic; some women simply can't grow enough follicles. From the extracted eggs, we were able get seven quality embryos. We decided to freeze two of the eggs for future use and have five implanted. We agreed not to do the FISH this time, as the doctors worried that it may have affected the last outcome. Obviously, implanting five embryos improved our odds for twins or triplets, and while that concerned us, having kids was more important. Doctors believe that multiple embryos assist each other to implant. The more helpers, the better the odds.

A week before getting our results, Andrea had some spotting. I wanted to run outside and scream as loud as I could, but Andrea stopped me. "Not so fast. I'm just spotting a little. This isn't like the first two times."

Andrea remembers that stressful time. "I had no clue if I was pregnant or not, but I knew that at that point Andy was pretty sure we weren't."

I stopped her by saying, "Let's not jinx it by talking about it further." But that night I prayed that we were pregnant. "God," I implored, "please let this be the one."

The fertility process had become tiresome. We'd spent a small fortune. Andrea had three surgical procedures and my testicles were becoming, well, testy. Emotionally, we were about a thousand miles past drained.

The dream of having kids was slowly disappearing for me. It seemed impossible. I was not going to watch my daughter's dance recitals or coach my son's baseball team. I began to wonder what I did that was so wrong. But while my dreams seemed to be slipping away, Andrea was having dreams that gave her confidence we might have a child.

More than once, we'd been asked by friends if we were trying to have kids. It was hard to respond to that, but Andrea came up with a good answer. "As you know, with Andy and me, it's not that easy. We can't have kids the fun way. It's a lot more work for us." That usually quieted those who were curious. But I was sick of having to answer the question that way. I wanted so much to shout the news from the rooftops: "Yes, we're pregnant!"

It seemed the day would never come, but finally it was time for Andrea to have the blood test to determine if she was pregnant. It had been two weeks since we started the shots. We would learn the results later that day.

Unlike the first two IVF attempts, Andrea had not gotten her period. I know because each time she went to the bathroom I'd ask, "Just some spotting, right? Nothing serious?" I'm sure it annoyed her, but I felt that if she had her period, I would at least know that we'd failed again. I tried to look for something to be positive about, but that's difficult during IVF.

That afternoon, I came home early and Andrea and I sat down to wait for the doctor's call. After a while, I went to Arby's to pick up a late lunch and, low and behold, the one near our house had closed. A bad omen? I wasn't sure. I went to another location and returned home with the food. We sat by the phone and looked at each other. My hands were shaking. I turned on the TV and found the movie *Sideways*. It seemed like hours passed, but it had only been thirty minutes. Then the phone rang.

Andrea picked up the receiver. False alarm, it was Andrea's dad. It rang again . . . my mom. Everyone wanted to know, but not as much as we did.

Andrea and I tried to be confident, but after back-to-back failures, it was difficult. Magic came over and put her head in each of our laps. It was as if she could tell what was happening. I then got a call on my cell. It was Nick Green's agent. Nick played for the Braves and his agent said Nick could come to A Wish for Wendy. Maybe that was the good omen we needed. I was reading omens into everything at this point. I even noticed that the antique table we ate our lunch on was the last keepsake I had from my granddad, Leon. Maybe his memory could bring us luck.

I started thinking what it would be like to have a child, but quickly stopped myself. I didn't want to think that far ahead. Andrea and I tried to talk about other things, but all we could think of was the news we were about to get. If it didn't work, would we resort to adopting or using a surrogate? Would we use someone else's sperm? Dr. Elsner told us we could find someone who looked like me and use his sperm. I was open to anything, but I wanted to give my own sperm a chance first.

Ringgggggggggggggggggggggg! Ringgggggggggggggggggggggg!

We looked at the caller ID and, sure enough, it was the doctor's office. We each took a deep breath. Andrea picked up the phone; it was Lynn, Dr. Elsner's nurse.

"Dr. Elsner would like to speak to you both," she said.

Andrea put us on speakerphone. Uh, oh, I thought. Usually, if a doctor personally wanted to talk, it meant bad news. At least that's what Andrea and I have noticed with all the calls we'd gotten over the past thirty years.

"Why, God? Why?" Andrea and I stared at each other and our heads began to droop as we waited to hear the news that seemed to be inevitable. Dr. Elsner probably wanted to discuss other options and give us an inspiring talk as to why we should not give up. As Dr. Elsner started to talk, I wiped the sweat from my forehead and hunched next to the phone.

"Andrea," she said, Dr. Elsner pronounced it "On-drea" so I always knew when she was on the phone. First, she asked how we were doing. It was like seeing the preview before a blockbuster movie you really wanted to see. "Get to it," I thought. "Well, guys . . ." She paused, "are you ready for the news? Andrea, my dear . . ." My heart was pumping so hard I thought it might jump from my chest and ricochet off our wall.

"You're pregnant!"

"What!" Andrea screamed. My heart somehow was able to beat even faster. One thought boomed in my head, "We're having a baby! We're having a baby! We're having a baby!" If I smoked cigars, I would have lit one right there. Darn CF again.

Andrea and I began to cry. Dr. Elsner said she doesn't usually call her patients with good news, but we were special. She wanted to be the one to tell us. Andrea recalls, "I remember being ecstatic at that point. I couldn't wait to tell my family and close friends. I then remember urinating on a stick just to see what a positive test result actually looked like."

I called my mom, then my dad. Then I called Emily, and Andrea called her brother, Alistair. When things settled down, I began to think of my sister, Wendy, who I knew must have seen how successful A Wish for Wendy had become. That success was my present to her and this, I believed, was her gift for me. It was then that I turned to Andrea and said, "We're having a girl!"

Andrea said, "We're not finding out until the baby is born."

"I already know," I told her. "We're having a beautiful baby girl."

Years later, I asked Dr. Elsner why our case meant so much to her. "Andy, you were the first cystic fibrosis patient I had worked with, and both you and Andrea are so loving and patient with the other. You both have good senses of humor. I never heard a cross word from either of you, even in the difficult times, and there was never a 'melt down' like we so frequently see when the going gets tough. You both were patient and persistent and I was not going to give up on you. I am ecstatic that it all worked out."

We were excited, too, but we had no idea what to expect next.

Chapter 34
A Difficult Pregnancy for Dad

Pregnancy was a scary time for us. Andrea and I had worked so hard to conceive and we just didn't want anything to go wrong. During the first trimester, Andrea and I went to the doctor to hear the baby's heartbeat. I was amazed. There was something alive in her stomach. I got teary eyed when I heard the baby's heartbeat for the first time. I couldn't stop listening. We decided that we needed a stress-reliever and Andrea had always wanted to go to Greece and Italy. Her father arranged a cruise for us. We were excited, but unfortunately we would never go on that trip.

I got a call from Andrea. "Honey, I am spotting. I am heading to my OB-GYN's office. Please come and meet me." I dropped the phone, grabbed my keys and sprinted to my car. Before I left, I made the mistake of telling someone at work that I had to leave because of an emergency with my wife. With my dad working in the company, of course, he heard. I drove down in a panic with the worst possible thoughts in mind. Were we losing the baby? Was Andrea's health in danger? Were we on the verge of disappointment yet again? I tried to remain calm. If not for my own sanity, I had to be collected for Andrea. Still, Andrea and I were terrified for the baby's health. We were at thirteen weeks and thought we were over the hump. Shortly after I arrived at Andrea's doctor's office, I got a call on my cell phone.

"Andy, it's Dad. Is Andrea okay?"

"Yes, she's fine."

"Can I see her?"

"Don't bother coming down, Dad. This place is forty-five minutes from work."

"Too late. I'm in the lobby."

Ten minutes later, my mom and sister followed through the same doors. Andrea's OB-GYN, Dr. Suarez, who had been seeing her since her college days at Emory, came out to get her and was surprised to see the waiting area filled with Lipmans. "Oh, the whole family is here," he smiled.

They did an ultrasound of Andrea's uterus and found some bleeding near the implantation site, but fortunately it had no effect on the baby. Eventually the bleeding stopped. That was the worst incident we had while Andrea was pregnant. The even better news was we got to hear the baby's heartbeat again and it was strong as ever. To me, that was the coolest part of pregnancy.

Still, the trip to the doctor scared me. It scared us both. Therefore, we decided to cancel the dream cruise to Greece and Italy. We didn't want to take the chance of having further issues and not being able to get proper medical attention.

We'd worked so hard to get pregnant. It had taken over a year. We'd spent a great deal of money, and we'd endured a lot of physical and emotional pain. I couldn't imagine how bad it would be if we lost the baby. I kept an eye on Andrea whenever I was near her. I protected her when I saw a potential accident—like water on the floor, or an extra step walking into a room. I didn't really get into watching or feeling the baby move inside Andrea's stomach. I thought it was more freaky than cool, and I worried when her stomach stopped moving that something might be wrong with the baby. When it came to my wife's expanding belly, I was always concerned about something. Growing up with cystic fibrosis and an over-protective mother probably caused me to be that way.

The next thing was coming up with a name. We had to use a name beginning with an "A," "E," "C," "W," or "L." In Jewish tradition, children are named after the first letter of a family member who has passed away. "A" would be after Andrea's maternal grandmother to whom she was very close. "E" and "L" were for my paternal grandparents. "C" was after my maternal grandfather. "W" was after Wendy.

With the infamous baby name book in hand, we began discussing potential baby names for baby Lipman, starting with a potential girl's name first—since I was so sure it was a girl.

"Allison," I said.

"It's a pretty name, but it just doesn't feel right," Andrea replied.

"Liz?" I blurted out.

"Honey, Liz Lipman? Do you want her to have a speech impediment?"

Finally I shouted out the last name of a former clutch pitcher for the Braves. It fit perfectly.

The boy's name took a while longer, although I was pretty sure it didn't matter. We were having a girl. I just knew it. Andrea thought we were having a boy and I'd heard that women usually have a sixth sense about this kind of thing. To this day, I don't know why I was so certain that we were having a girl. I just was.

Months went by. I had a work trip to Chicago two weeks before the due date and I was worried I'd miss the birth due to the snow falling in Chicago. Some of our friends, whose due dates were later, had already had their babies.

It was frustrating. Every time we visited the doctor, his answer was the same, "I don't see any dilation."

As Valentine's Day drew closer, we worried that if we had a girl she'd be miserable if her birthday was on Valentine's Day. I've been told that from a girl's perspective, it's the worst. On Valentine's Day night, Andrea and I drove to Bucca di Beppo, hoping the baby would arrive soon. We almost tried the eggplant, which is known to have a good effect on labor, but we weren't quite that desperate yet. After all, our due date was either February 14th or February 17th, depending on which doctor was asked. That night, it took the waitress over an hour to get our food. I finally grabbed the manager and said, "I have a very pregnant wife, it's Valentine's Day, and our food hasn't shown up in over an hour." We ended up getting a free meal but still no baby!

On Friday morning, February 17, 2006, I had just woken up when Andrea called me to the bathroom to see something. "Honey," she whispered, "my mucous plug came out." She almost seemed like she enjoyed looking at this disgusting white blob of mucous in our toilet. I guess that was the scientist in her. Seeing the mucous plug didn't give me the same satisfaction that it gave my wife, but I knew what its presence meant. It was pretty much the only thing I remembered from our birthing class, other than the fact that the ceiling in the classroom had two hundred and twelve tiles. While this could mean the baby might come in the next few hours, we might still be days away. Either way, we had to be prepared. Andrea's contractions began at ten minutes apart and were growing more regular by the hour. I remembered being a kid and watching *The Flintstones* episode when Wilma went into labor with Pebbles. Fred freaked out and grabbed the suitcase, but forgot his wife on the way to the hospital. I was a little calmer.

We left for the doctor's office and on the way called to tell our parents to stand-by. Fortunately, we had an appointment with Dr. Suarez that day so he had availability to see us at eleven A.M. After our examination, the doctor looked at Andrea and said, "You're dilated three centimeters and contractions are only three minutes apart. You're having a baby today."

Andrea wanted to have a natural birth. She was doing great with the contractions. She was not experiencing much pain at all.

Andrea reminisces: "How easy is this?" I thought. "I'd seen all of these labor videos and thought I was going to be screaming in tremendous pain. I was just fine."

Then the doctor wanted to speed things up so he came in and broke her water himself. That's when things took a turn. Andrea's contractions got more intense. "They intensified one thousand-fold!" she remembers. It was difficult to watch her go through it. It was like a trainer watching his boxer get destroyed in the ring but there's nothing he can do to stop the fight. Andrea was squeezing my finger so tight, it nearly broke. After thirty minutes of excruciating pain, Andrea succumbed and requested an epidural and that's when things got strange.

The anesthesiologist apparently was having a bad day. When he walked in and asked if we were ready, the nurse said, "Give us one minute. We are in the middle of a contraction." Andrea screamed in pain.

"I'll go then. Call me when she's ready," he said, as if we had insulted him.

"Just give us a second and we'll be ready," the nurse repeated.

"You're not ready. I'll come back!" he said angrily as he shut the door.

I thought this was some sort of joke. What kind of medical professional walks out on his patient? The nurse raced after him in embarrassment. He finally came back and gave her the epidural. She felt some immediate relief, but was now confined to the bed since the lower part of her body was numb. Finally, at six P.M., Dr. Suarez said it was time to push.

After two hours—and a lot of hard work on Andrea's part—the doctor said, "The baby's head is too big, and I'm concerned the baby may be turned the wrong way. We're going to need to do a C-section."

Andrea was disappointed, as she'd been standing on the bed tightly gripping a push bar for the last two hours, while being essentially numb from the waist down. She'd wanted more than anything to push that baby out. She was also nervous for obvious reasons, but she was assured there was no other way. The family, already there and waiting, was concerned. But I told them it would all be fine and to be excited. In the next thirty minutes, they were going to be grandparents, and Andrea and I... well, we were going to be parents!

I was remarkably calm, but I'm not sure why. Normally, when things are stressful, I freak out. Not this time. I had a beautiful wife, a great family, and soon, a beautiful daughter . . . wink, wink.

They took Andrea to the operating room and I was escorted to a temporary private room where I immediately called Ross to tell him that in a matter of minutes I was going to be a dad. Moments later, as I looked at myself in the mirror in mustard yellow surgical garb, a tall surgeon came in and asked if I was ready. He sounded like we were going to a football game rather than my kid's birth. "You ready, Mr. Lipman? Here we go!"

The first thing I saw when I walked in was a lot of blood. I thought I was going to faint, but as soon as I saw Andrea's face, I wanted to comfort her. "It's okay," I told her definitively. "It's going to be all right." She was shaking and sweating and looking very scared, but then she smiled. The last two years had been so difficult, but the next moments made it all worthwhile.

When the doctors pulled out a crying baby, it took a second to dawn on me that the inconsolable infant was my child. The moment was surreal—like I was watching all this happen to someone else. As the screams became louder, I worried about the baby's health, but I was assured that this was normal. At least I knew that, unlike me, this kid's lungs were in great shape.

I took a picture at the very first moment of birth. Then I got a great picture of Andrea seeing the baby for the first time. One of the doctors got a kick out of asking if I wanted to see Andrea's uterus.

"No thanks," I said, wondering if he was serious.

The baby was beautiful. The nurses cleared the nostrils and checked the vital signs. Everything looked great. I flashed more pictures; I was a proud papa.

Our baby was eight pounds, three ounces, had blonde hair and blue eyes and was born just after nine that night. I'm a numbers guy, so I immediately tried to figure out the number significance of the birth. The baby was born 02/17/06. Wendy passed away 01/02/71. Both dates had two zeros, a one, and a seven. The only numbers left were a one and a six. Wendy lived sixteen days.

The baby was a spitting image of me, from eye color to skin complexion. It was almost frightening how much we looked alike. As they put the baby in the rolling little bed, I left Andrea momentarily and headed toward the nursery where my parents, Aunt Susie, Andrea's father, and Nana were waiting to see our family's newest member. Andrea's mother was in California. She and her husband caught the first flight and would arrive the following morning. Emily was away at school, and Alistair lived on the west coast, so they would meet our new addition shortly thereafter.

It was time to announce the news. "Everybody," I jubilantly yelled, "meet your new granddaughter, Avery Leah Lipman."

Thank you, Wendy, for a beautiful baby girl.

She was *A.L.L.* we'd ever wanted.

Chapter 35
Parenting CF Style

The best analogy I ever heard about life before and after having a child illustrates it with a pay-inside gas station visit. Without a child you just pumped the gas, walked into the station, paid, got in the car and drove off. With a child, you pump the gas, check on the baby, pick up her pacifier, talk to her, unbuckle her seatbelt, take her out, check if her diaper is heavy, find a spot to change her diaper, make her stop crying, walk inside with her, try to open your wallet with one hand while still holding her with the other, fumble around for cash or a credit card, pay, go back to your car, put her back in the seat, tighten the belt, give her a toy, go around, get in, start the car, hit your head on the steering wheel, and finally drive away. Hitting your head on the steering wheel is optional, but it works for me.

When Andrea and I brought Avery home for the first time, we were nervous wrecks. I will admit I was glad to leave the hospital, not because of the germs, but because I was tired of sleeping in a chair that felt more like a coffin. We'd been there for three nights. It was comforting that several of our friends were also there delivering babies. It was kind of like a tight-knit fraternity.

I was afraid to drive home because I didn't want to get in an accident with the baby in the car. Andrea was just scared. Her life, more than mine, had completely changed. She was now responsible for breastfeeding every three hours, changing a lot of diapers, soothing a crying infant, and she'd have to decide if she was going back to work.

Avery tested negative for cystic fibrosis, which was something that made me very happy. The odds were very slim, but I still worried. She will be a carrier, but my hope is that it won't matter in twenty-five years because there will be a cure.

Unfortunately, Avery did not come with instructions, but we found a great doula. A doula is a caregiver who visits the first week the baby comes home and teaches new parents how to care for their baby. She also organizes the house so things are easy to find. Mostly, she makes the transition from carefree person to instant parent a lot easier.

We also found Luz, a great nanny who began working for us when Avery was four months old. She comes five times a week and that allowed Andrea to go back to work at the CDC. Avery loves Luz. They sing and dance and she's taught Avery a second language, Spanish. Oh, and she loves putting Avery's hair in pigtails. It's the cutest thing ever.

As far as having cystic fibrosis and a baby, I've had to make adjustments. Instead of working out at night, I save that time to spend with Avery. I leave work early two days a week, and I work out and do my therapy in the morning so I can help Andrea when Avery wakes up. We both have to get ready for work so we take turns watching her. Andrea has been an amazing mother. Pumping milk three or four times a day every day for more than a year was one of the most difficult logistical tasks she has ever faced. It was frustrating— and Andrea didn't love doing it—but she knew it was the best way for the baby to get disease-fighting antibodies.

I initially put my medications on the top shelf of our closet so Avery could not reach them. We eventually invested in a medicine cabinet with a lock and key, which we still keep on the top shelf. From the start, I've had a fear that she might swallow some of my pills. I will say that she is sometimes curious about the vibrating vest I use to do my therapy. She stands up and leans against it so she shakes too. Then she taps on it as if we're playing Hide-and-Seek. Still for the most part, I can tell that she's a bit afraid of it and that is probably because she's rarely up with me at five in the morning when I'm doing my therapy.

The hardest times for me are those moments when I worry about getting deadly bacteria or dying at an early age. I don't want to leave Avery. I want to do so many things with her, but I also know that my life and health are vulnerable. Many of my guy friends don't go to their kids' music classes or birthday parties. I do, because I don't know how much time I'll have with my daughter and I want to make the most of every moment. Maybe I'm lucky in that regard. I realize that life is short and I'm making the most of it. My daughter is going to remember her father.

Avery is just beautiful. She favors me a lot, but she makes those looks work. So far her hair has stayed blonde, though it looks as if it will turn brown someday. She kept her blue eyes, has a beautiful smile, and a laugh that makes me want to grab her and tickle her all over.

She's pretty smart, too. She walked at nine months. Nine months! I walked much later than that, but Andrea was an early walker. Avery also learned to sign a few words so that we could understand her before she could talk clearly. She started talking around a year old.

She loves to play basketball. At eleven months, I taught her how to dribble, well, at least pat the ball. She also loves to play ping pong, pinball, pool, Centipede and Galaga. That's our entire basement collection. We got her involved in soccer when she was three but she didn't favor it, even though I coached her team. At four, she really got involved in gymnastics, which has become her sport of choice. She's already getting recognition as one of the better gymnasts in her class. Watch out, Mary Lou Retton!

I'm not one of those parents who is determined his kid will be a megastar athlete, but I want her to enjoy sports. I learned so many things from sports—including how to be a good teammate, how to sacrifice for others and how to expect success from myself. When she starts beating me, then we might have a problem. Magic and Avery get along great, too. I was told that if you take a blanket your baby used at the hospital and let your dog sleep with it, there will be an instant bond between the two. I had my doubts, but I tried it and the moment Avery came home, Magic sniffed her and went about her business.

Avery and Magic have a routine. Avery drops whatever food she doesn't want and Magic eats it. Magic lies under her seat like a vulture waiting for prey. At night, Magic rewards Avery for her generosity by sleeping next to her door.

Seeing the two of them together brought tears to my eyes because it reminded me of the days Howard and I ran around the house together. Dogs are amazing companions and I am happy that Avery is growing up with one of the best.

I'm thrilled to have Avery in my life. I'm charmed by the way she says "Daddy!" and runs and jumps in my arms. It truly is the best feeling I can imagine. I am so very grateful for her because she is something I never thought I could have.

Chapter 36
A Normal Day at the Doctor's Office

Even though both Andrea and I had been focused on the pregnancy, neither of us had forgotten about my health issues. Going to the doctor's office for a check-up is not a big deal for most people, but my situation, obviously, is different.

In the past, I would have to pack my meds, fly out to Cincinnati, Ohio and visit Dr. Boat, whom I'd been seeing since the tenth grade. There were several downfalls to flying to my doctor's appointments. First, I had to make sure my pills, frozen medication, and therapy equipment were properly packed. It's not like a forgotten hairbrush that I can buy when I get to Cincinnati. My medication is very unusual and from the wrong pharmacy, it can be quite expensive.

Then there is the issue with carrying all of my CF stuff through the airport. After about fifteen minutes of carrying the therapy machine, the strap would begin to dig into my shoulder pretty badly leaving long red marks on my skin. I never check my therapy or aerosol machine bags because of all the medications. I didn't want any of it to be lost. After ticketing, I had to go straight to security, which became a bottleneck when I got to the front of the line.

When I put my bags through the checker, all the security people looked on the screen and then looked at each other. Then they grabbed the bag, and I raised my hand before I even knew which bag they're grabbing. "That's mine," I laughed.

From the navy blue bag, they would pull out a white machine that looks like a boom box radio. But if this machine were to break, it would cost about five thousand times more than a radio. After rubbing a pad all over it, they would seal it back up. Then they would look in the black bag, which stores my aerosol machine. After they checked that, I showed them the note from my doctor, which allowed me to carry an ice pack and my frozen meds in a cooler bag. Currently, passengers are not allowed to carry an icepack on board without written authorization.

About ten minutes later, I would finally be cleared to go and make the walk with all my stuff to the gate. Upon arrival, I carry my stuff through the

Cincinnati airport, get a rental car, drive to my hotel and then shortly after, to my appointment with Dr. Boat.

Dr. Boat has known me longer than my wife, most of my close friends, and almost as many years as my sister, Emily. In the time since Dr. Boat started treating me, I've gone from being a bony teenager, who'd accomplished very little, to a muscular young man who has a job, a family and who regularly plays tennis, softball and basketball.

It was stressful enough just having a doctor's appointment. The hard work to get there did nothing for my pulmonary function scores. In the last few years, I found a doctor at Emory University only thirty minutes from my home. Deciding not to see Dr. Boat anymore was difficult. I knew that I would miss him and the banter we used to have. We used to argue less about my health but more about who was the better team: his Cincinnati Reds or my Atlanta Braves. Still, it was time. I knew that by the new patches of grey in his beard and the fact that he was seeing far fewer patients that Dr. Boat was getting older and he would soon retire. I still trusted him with my health and asked that any doctor who worked with me to consult him before giving me any new meds.

At Emory, I originally worked with Dr. Arlene Stecenko and then Dr. Lindy Wolfenden, a young, bright doctor whose knowledge and passion reminded me so much of Dr. Boat. When we met, Dr. Wolfenden was in her late thirties and had curly brown hair and a vivacious smile. She had a great sense of humor, as well, which she needed to understand my wit. She became as much a friend as a doctor.

The night prior to each check-up seems as if I'm preparing to be called to war. I get calls of encouragement from several of my good friends, my Aunt Susie, Nana Rose and, of course, my mom and dad. They call to tell me that everything is going to be fine; these calls help set the tone for my journey. Andrea always hugs and kisses me and reminds me to call her as soon as my appointment is over to let her know how I'm doing.

I have grown accustomed to going to the doctor on my own. I used to go with my mom, but I angered her with my tirade in college when we saw Dr. Boat at the University of North Carolina. I have also gone with my father, and Andrea has gone with me as well, but, to be honest, I like going by myself because I develop a warrior's mentality when I walk through the electric doors of the hospital. I'm always nervous for my appointments. Heck, I usually fret about it for a couple of weeks before I go. But when I walk through those hospital doors, you'd never know that I was scared. I treat my doctor's appointment like it is a sport. It is me against CF, and I relish the challenge.

Sometimes the doctor asks that I get a chest X-ray. I remember when I was in my early thirties and still at the University of Cincinnati and walking up to the Children's Hospital radiology receptionist and having her ask, "Where is Andrew?" It seemed to be a different person each time but the conversation was always the same.

"I'm him. Expecting someone a bit younger?" It never failed. They always thought I was the father and not the patient. To be fair, though, I was easily the oldest patient there. The sad thing was I saw a lot of babies waiting their turn. Seeing all the kids in wheelchairs or with oxygen tanks was the most unsettling part of visiting a children's hospital. Now, CF patients are living longer, so it's less of a surprise when someone with CF, who also happens to be in his mid-thirties, requests an X-ray.

While at my doctor's appointments, I do the "normal" stuff. I get my weight, blood pressure and temperature checked. Then when my nurse, Welela Berhanu, whom I've been seeing at Emory for more than three years, is done recording my stats, she asks what medications I am currently taking. I used to ask if she was subject to writer's cramp because the list was so long. The first time I listed my meds, she was sweating and using the back of the page to write it all down. Now they keep a list of my meds on the computer so Welela has a much easier time updating my list of daily, weekly and monthly intake of drugs. After a brief discussion about how I was doing, Welela leaves and I meet with my dietician, Jessica Enders. She and I go over my diet and ways to improve my eating habits. Then I am greeted by my PFT (pulmonary function test) administrator, Mews Hilaire, who tests my breathing. This is by far the scariest, yet most exhilarating, activity I do at my doctor's appointments.

If my function goes down, there are big concerns. If it stays the same or goes up, I can boast of my success. When it comes to my PFT numbers, I'm as competitive as anyone, but with PFTs, being competitive is a good thing. I compete against my previous numbers and I set high standards for myself.

I joke with Mews about one thing or another, just to keep the mood light. Since I was young, I've used comedy to break up the seriousness of cystic fibrosis. In a way, humor has been my self-defense mechanism. If I think about how serious and scary CF is, I'll put a lot of pressure on myself. The looser I am, the better I perform. In some ways, comedy is like my therapy machine. While my machine breaks up the mucous in my lungs so I can breathe, my humor breaks up the seriousness in the room—so I can breathe.

I grab a tube and put it between my teeth and lips for the PFT, then put a clothes-pin-like device on my nose so that I can only breathe through my mouth. I sit in the chair and adjust the tube. I think about Wendy and Andrea as sources of motivation, take three easy breaths, then a big breath, and blow as hard as I can. My goal is to get most of the numbers above 90 percent. The percentages compare me to the average person, not just to those with cystic fibrosis. It's nice to have great numbers on the first turn because it relieves some of the pressure, but also because it only gets tougher after that. Each time I take the test, Mews screams, "Blow! Blow! Blow!" And when I run out of air he shouts, "Inhale as fast as you can."

Next, I wait for Dr. Wolfenden to come in so we can examine my PFT scores and any other tests that I may have had that day. Other tests I take annually are bone density tests to examine the strength of my bones and glucose tests, which is a test that requires taking more than a dozen vials of my blood to see if I have diabetes. CF patients are more likely than most to get diabetes. In fact, we have our own diabetes called cystic fibrosis-related diabetes or CFRD. It's not something we brag about. CFRD is found in more than 40 percent of CF patients above the age of thirty. I have yet to be diagnosed with it. Unfortunately, my bone density test detected that I have osteopenia, which means I'm on the verge of having osteoporosis. Therefore, as if I didn't take enough drugs already, the doctor had to add several calcium tablets a day.

Chapter 37
Getting the Picture

Shortly after Avery's birth, I was called by WXIA, Atlanta's NBC affiliate. "You've been nominated for a community service award by your aunt, Susie Davis. You are one of our eleven recipients. Would you be willing to accept this honor?"

I had no idea that I was nominated and I honestly had never heard of the CSAs (Community Service Awards). Andrea, my parents, and Aunt Susie all knew about it, but didn't want to tell me in case I didn't win. I was going to speak on television!

Over the years, I had spoken to many groups about my story in hopes of raising awareness about cystic fibrosis research. In 2002 I was honored to be asked to give the closing speech at the Center for Disease Control and Prevention's Center for Birth Defects and Developmental Disabilities conference. Dana Reeve, wife of the late Christopher Reeve, also spoke, which made me feel I was in good company.

A month after I got the call about winning the Community Service Award, a cameraman from the station came to my house. He filmed me working out, doing my therapy, and running. He filmed our little baby girl and introduced us to Paul Ossmann, WXIA's meteorologist. I didn't know much about Paul, but he'd been there to ease my fears in years past about the weather for A Wish for Wendy. It was good to find that Paul was as genuine as they come. He brought his son, Grant, along because he was a huge baseball fan and he'd heard I was, too. I showed Grant my baseball memorabilia collection and Paul and I talked baseball trivia for more than an hour. We went to the tennis courts in my neighborhood and filmed an exhibition between Paul and me. He was okay, but I could tell he hadn't played in several years.

Toward the end of our filming, the cameraman asked if we had a picture of Wendy. I had never asked my mom to see her picture because I was afraid it was too personal. But, I decided this was a chance for all of Atlanta to see the inspiration for our fight. Mom was at my house helping with Avery so I asked her, "Do you still have the picture of Wendy?" There was only one picture. It was a black and white picture taken by my parents' friends, Bill and

Sandee Carlisle, just before my sister was whisked away from my mom's arms at the hospital.

Mom ran home and retrieved the cherished photograph from the bottom of a drawer. For the first time, I saw the person for whom I'd tried so hard to grant a wish. She looked just as I thought she would: dark hair, pale skin, and features a bit like Avery's. I took a few minutes to look at her, and in my mind I told her, "It's all for you."

In April, I went to the WXIA *11 Alive* studio, where the eleven CSA recipients met each other. Each of these individuals had their own amazing story. It reminded me a lot of running with the Olympic Torch. Three stories stood out: a student at the University of Georgia who ran a program for mentally challenged children; a man and his wife who had their own adaptive learning center where they helped children with developmental disabilities get adopted; and a woman in her eighties who helped provide food for seniors to improve their day-to-day lives.

Before we spoke, there was a two-minute segment on each of us that we would not see until it aired. My piece featured a person from the Cystic Fibrosis Foundation talking about me. It showed me playing softball and tennis, and included a close-up of Andrea and me with Avery. At the end was the picture of Wendy, so everyone could see our inspiration for the softball tournament.

The recipients had been told we had only forty-five seconds to speak. How could I tell my life story in forty-five seconds? For a week I pondered, then wrote:

> I wasn't supposed to be here today. I wasn't supposed to be here ten years ago or even twenty, but thanks to the funds donated to the Cystic Fibrosis Foundation, I'm not just living; I'm thriving.
>
> I want to thank my father, Charles Lipman, for his love and support; my mom, Eva, and my Aunt Susie for nominating me; the love of my life, Andrea, who is a fighter in her own right; my sister Emily; and my seven-week old daughter, Avery, who doctors told me I could never have.
>
> While working on the filming of my story, I was able to see a picture of my sister, Wendy, for the first time. I dedicate this award to Wendy. Although her short life was truly tragic, her spirit continues to be magic.
>
> Please come out to Alpharetta's North Park on November 4th so you too can contribute to the magic we call A Wish for Wendy.
>
> Thank you.

When I finished, I got a big hand from the people in attendance. Josh and several other friends were able to join my parents and Andrea for the special occasion. I also posed for a picture with Atlanta Falcons' defensive-end Patrick Kerney, who towered above me. Four days later, the show aired. I watched it with Andrea, my parents, Emily, and Nana Rose.

All and all, it was a true success. A lot of money was raised for charity and A Wish for Wendy was given one thousand dollars from *11 Alive* in gratitude for what we had done. Paul Ossmann came to A Wish for Wendy as a celebrity coach, and his team won the whole thing. Paul and I still keep in touch via e-mail, and he brings Grant to every Wish for Wendy. I'm very glad I made a friend from the experience.

I've mentioned the dream where a girl finds me under a clothes rack in a department store. Just after my twenty-fifth birthday I figured out the girl was Wendy. Seven years later, I no longer had the dream about Wendy and I wondered if realizing it was her was all she wanted me to know. Yet, I felt as though something were still missing. During the Community Service Awards, I finally was able to see her picture. About a year after that, Wendy came to visit one final time.

I went to bed early that night, and since Avery was finally sleeping through the night, I was sleeping really well. In my dream I found myself in a classroom. The classroom was completely white, except for a green chalkboard a few feet behind the teacher. The teacher, an older lady with thick glasses and gray hair, was talking, but I could not comprehend anything she said. I didn't know any of the students and couldn't understand anything. I felt stupid. It was as if I'd been absent all semester and was suddenly thrown in this class and had to catch up with everyone else.

I started to panic when a finger tapped my right shoulder. I turned around and there she was. My little sister had grown up. Wendy was now in her thirties, as she actually would have been. She had long brown hair, dark brown eyes and a look of calmness that I so badly needed to see. She looked at me, but did not say a word. Then Wendy's lips curled, but this was no ordinary smile. It was the warmest smile I'd ever seen. Immediately I woke up.

I didn't figure out the dream until weeks later, after I had a chance to think about it. All my life I had trouble understanding why I lived and Wendy died. Nor did I understand why I wanted so much to do something for someone I'd never met. Why did the fundraising idea come to me? Why was A Wish for Wendy so successful? Why have so many good things happened to me over the years? Compared to most people with CF, I rarely got sick. I'd been able to stave off infections for the most part. Why?

Then I thought back to the dream. While I could not understand the teacher, the girl behind me understood everything and reassured me that it would be okay. She's always been behind me, though most of the time I haven't known. I thought the teacher represented life. How was I still alive and thriving despite having a disease that took most people as young children? I never knew what to do, but behind me sat the student who understood everything. She was the one who would inspire her younger brother to make a difference against cystic fibrosis. She was behind many of my decisions when it came to CF.

I never had that dream again and, in the last few years, my sister has not been a part of any of my dreams. I truly believe that was her last message to me. It's hard to imagine that I can miss someone I never met, yet I miss her terribly. It comforts me to believe that she grows up each day as I do, just in a different place, and that she's happy for what we've accomplished with A Wish for Wendy. One day, I'll visit her classroom again and maybe she'll tell me why she was taken so early in life and why I was given the opportunity to live. One day, we'll have that longed-for brother-sister chat.

Chapter 38
Trying for Baby Number Two

In August of 2007, Andrea and I decided it was time to try again. We both wanted two children. To be honest, I was thrilled just to have one, but I wanted Avery to have a sibling. Okay, I also wanted a second child—I wanted to experience the moment of welcoming a baby, my baby, into the world again. It was wonderful.

Andrea and I were both thirty-four years old and, statistically, for a woman, it starts to become more difficult to have children after thirty-five. We had frozen two embryos the last time we were at "Club 1150" and we hadn't been back in more than two years. Now we were starting the process again. After a month of shots for Andrea, plus progesterone injections during the last week, we were ready for implantation. First however, the doctors had to see if either of the embryos was viable when they were thawed.

At our appointment the nurse practitioner told us that only one embryo had survived the thaw. It was a four-cell embryo, which was not ideal. The doctors were hoping for one with six to eight-cells. Our odds of conceiving were significantly lower with only one embryo to implant but not completely impossible. Dr. Elsner told us of many miracle cases where the odds were far less than ours, but she refused to give percentages. The doctors transferred the embryo into Andrea, but not before I showed off my latest pictures of Avery. It was interesting to see how proud they were of our little girl. The doctors acted as if she were their child, too. Avery truly became part of a big family there. She was one of the ones who made it.

Since the procedure took three tries and five embryos last time, I didn't have a good reason to be optimistic, but I hated for Andrea to have all the shots needed for repeated implantations. If this attempt failed she would have to go through that and a lot more.

After the implant I went to work and Andrea went home to relax, which meant relaxing for the next few weeks if we were going to be successful. My cousin and his wife had just had a baby, but we could not go to the bris, as I was still administering Andrea's shots and Avery had an ear infection.

Plus, Nana had just broken her arm at synagogue so my mother rushed to Charleston to help care for her.

I was having dreams every night. The first night, I dreamt we got the call that we were pregnant. The second night, the procedure did not work. The third night we already had the baby. It was maddening to wake up and know there was still another week before we'd know anything.

As the time for the end of Andrea's monthly cycle loomed closer, she said, "I hope I don't get my period in the next few days." I told her I didn't want to think that far ahead, though I'd been thinking about it days before she even mentioned it. I'm not sure which is worse: the physical strain going through fertility puts on a couple or the emotional distress.

Throughout the week, I asked Andrea if she felt like she was pregnant. "In some ways, yes, and in some ways, no," she said.

I kept asking for signs. I know I was looking for a reason to stay motivated, despite knowing I had to hurt Andrea everyday with the shots and it could all be for nothing. What stung most was that nearly all people get pregnant easily and some not even on purpose. I wished we could be like most couples and have a baby the fun way.

The drugs affected Andrea's emotions and the shot-giving procedure put me on edge. We bickered more than we ordinarily did, mostly about unimportant things.

I wanted very much for this to be the last time we'd have to go through IVF treatments. Andrea's hip was red from the shots and she was itching badly. It wasn't fair.

Then as the days got closer, she said, "Maybe I am pregnant. I haven't had my period, yet." But her periods had been late several times over the last few months so that didn't keep me from worrying. I thought her breasts looked bigger, which was a sign of pregnancy, but the meds she was on also augmented breast size.

As D-Day (Discovery Day) approached, I asked Andrea after every morning bathroom episode if she had bled at all and, up till then, she had not. I couldn't stand the wait anymore. I'd counted down the number of mornings and the number of shots I had to give before we got an answer. It was draining. I was trying not to get my hopes up. After all, the odds were slim at best.

Two nights before we found out, Andrea told me that her side was really hurting. She didn't know if it was her ovaries before her period came, or possibly an ectopic pregnancy. I wouldn't want it to be either, but an ectopic pregnancy (meaning a fertilized egg has implanted outside of the uterus) would be especially bad, because it would require surgery to remove it. Andrea researched her symptoms on the Internet. She was always curious to know why her body reacted in certain ways. I, on the other hand, preferred not knowing. The next day I attended the Georgia game with some friends who already had kids. They asked me if I was ready for another. "Not thinking about it right now," I said, which wasn't a total lie, since I was trying to clear my head and enjoy the game.

The attempts to keep IVF a secret reminded me of a speech I gave to a Rotary Club around that time. I talked about what going through IVF was like. Most of these men were older and probably didn't know the first thing about fertility procedures. When I was done, a young club member tapped me on the shoulder and whispered, "So you go to RBA? Who is your doctor?" Turns out there are a lot more people going through this than I thought.

D-Day arrived with no blood for Andrea. I was slightly optimistic. We'd played a Ping-Pong game so we wouldn't think about the call. We had just begun watching Goonies on HBO when the phone rang. Caller ID showed it was our neighbor, so we let the phone ring.

When the phone rang again, it was the clinic. I crossed my fingers. In fact, I was sweating profusely just waiting for the news. "Hi guys, it's Lynn." I could tell by her voice that the procedure had probably failed. "Well, I don't have good news." She asked how we were doing and told us to call Dr. Elsner and set up a conference call.

I didn't think I'd be so disappointed, but I was. I really was. Andrea took it a lot better than I did. She was disappointed, of course, but she was already mentally preparing herself for our next attempt. Friends had told me that once you had a child that it was easier to take a failed attempt, but I didn't feel that way. Maybe it was knowing we'd have to start all over again. Maybe it was knowing that the sole reason why we'd have to go through the shots and procedures again was because of my inadequacies. Maybe I was concerned because Andrea was growing closer to thirty-five, and as each month went by it was only going to be harder to have children. I wasn't devastated, but I was deeply disappointed. Then Avery in her freshly bathed pigtails ran into the room and gave me a big hug, not knowing it was the best medicine she could give me.

"Daddy!" she said, "Daddy, hello!"

Then I saw the big picture. Thank goodness we used her embryo when we did. It probably would not have worked if we'd frozen it and used it alone. It confirmed to me that little Avery was a miracle, and instead of dwelling on what we did not have, it was time I appreciated the beautiful girl we did have.

A few days later, Andrea and I had a conference call with Dr. Elsner. We spoke about the disappointment of not being pregnant and also of our excitement to try again. We knew that the next time around we'd have a better opportunity. For one, the doctor was going to put us back on the flare protocol that helped us have Avery, and we wouldn't be using frozen embryos. Andrea was also making appointments for acupuncture, which some said helped achieve conception.

Our only concern was that Andrea's mom was having a big Thanksgiving in Florida, because Andrea's brother was coming to town. We didn't get many chances to see Alistair, so we really wanted to go. Had Andrea's cycle been regular, we'd have had no problem going to Florida; however, her periods seemed to run a little later every month. There was a chance that the implanting would happen around the time we were supposed to leave. At that time a Thanksgiving vacation was not our number one priority. We also knew that if this procedure failed, the doctors would have to re-evaluate the situation and we'd have to wait months to try again.

Andrea and I began our second attempt a few weeks later. We'd be undergoing surgical procedures again to produce the embryos. By this time we knew we'd be missing Thanksgiving. In vitro pretty much puts life on hold. Planning trips, get-togethers with friends or even a nice dinner becomes secondary. You just don't know how the schedule is going to pan out.

Early one morning in late November of 2007, we arrived at "Club 1150" and Andrea was taken into surgery two hours later. Then I noticed something I hadn't noticed in the past. The surgical area was on the sixth floor. The number six had always been my lucky number. Maybe it could be lucky one more time.

After picking up Andrea's pain meds, I spoke with Dr. Elsner, who was pleased with the results of the surgery. "We got twelve eggs," she said. That was similar to our first attempt with Avery, but again, quantity didn't matter, quality did, and we wouldn't know the quality until we had the transfer.

Next, I was told to put on my hospital garb, which included a backless gown and brown socks with sticky plastic on the bottoms so I wouldn't slip. Dr. Witt was not there, yet, so I waited as Andrea dozed in the post-op room. She and I talked a little, but she was still groggy. She asked if I was ready for Tom Selleck, her little joke that Dr. Witt looked like the *Magnum, P.I* star. I went through two *People* magazines before he arrived from a surgery at another building.

I reminded Dr. Witt about using the right testicle last time and he said, "Yeah, that was the successful one." The first needle stung, but, once numb, I only felt pulls and tugs, not sharp pain. Dr. Witt and I talked about Avery, Andrea, and some of the things going on in the world, which helped take my mind off what was happening.

Before leaving, I had our nurse put targets on Andrea's hips so I could aim the shot. It's easier when they show me exactly where the shots should go. This time, for some reason, the circles were much smaller. Had the circles been too big previously?

We began our shots the next night. Our previous order did not have sesame oil. When we got pregnant with Avery, we used injections with sesame oil so it made sense to use that medication again. I hoped that wasn't the reason for the last failure. On the second night I put the shot in before the alcohol had a chance to dry. It stung Andrea and her squeal of pain really stung me. Hearing my best friend cry because of something I did was awful. The worst part was that I had to get beyond it and do it the next night and the next and the next.

The following day was bad, too. Andrea took my car to Avery's gym class and, as luck would have it, the transmission went out, stranding them on the side of the road. It was the first time my 4Runner had ever died. Andrea was on so many hormonal drugs that she was crying on the phone. Thank goodness my aunt lived nearby and was able to help. I hoped this was not the same kind of omen we'd had when Possum died.

That Sunday, we went for the transfer. We were excited that they told us to come in because it meant at least one embryo was viable. We were not allowed to wear perfume, deodorant or any other type of scented product because it could affect the embryos. I didn't want to take any chances, so I didn't even brush my teeth. We were told that nine eggs matured and six fertilized, which was a pretty good number. The big question was how many of the fertilized eggs were actually quality embryos.

Andrea was not allowed to go to the bathroom until after the transfer, so she had to hold her bladder for several hours, plus drink lots of water so they could see everything in the ultrasound. When the nurse was done checking to make sure that Andrea's bladder was full, she turned on the monitor, which showed how many embryos were available. Andrea predicted we'd have four, but she actually thought we'd have three. I didn't guess, as I was too nervous.

I held Andrea's hand, closed my eyes and prayed. The screen flashed on and five embryos appeared. Andrea and I thought it was karma. The five embryos looked exactly the same as those when we were successful with Avery. The embryo specialist was a little apprehensive but after looking at our chart, he agreed with us that all five embryos needed to be implanted. Andrea was excited about having five. I felt bad that I was so nonchalant, but I didn't want to get too excited. I'd been disappointed in the past. I also knew the outcome was something I could not control, and my attitude had little to do with our chances of success.

That afternoon, Andrea went home and rested. She was not allowed to lift Avery for at least twenty-four hours, so I took Avery to a birthday party at a place called Monkey Joe's, where kids can jump on bouncy toys. Everyone asked where Andrea was and I told them she was feeling under the weather. I hoped no one thought that meant she was pregnant. That was my worst fear, because there was a very real chance she wasn't.

Over the next few weeks we tried to think about other things, but it was difficult. I focused on looking for a new car or buying Hanukkah gifts—anything but IVF. Every night, Andrea and I talked to our embryos after we did the shot. "Implant," we begged. "Implant!" We added the pictures of our embryos to the pictures of our Dave & Buster's kids and the pictures of our embryos that produced Avery. We still played our eighties music. We felt our odds were better because Andrea had done acupuncture this time, we had more embryos, and they were in better condition. Still, it was a crapshoot.

I tried to think of the positives. We had a beautiful baby girl. We had a nice house, good jobs, and even though I have CF and Andrea has MS, our health was relatively good. But I kept returning to thoughts of having another baby. After implanting, there were fourteen more injections until we knew the results. Friday the 14th could not arrive fast enough.

A week before we'd find out, we got some terrible news. Andrea called me at work and said something awful had happened. I knew she'd been crying.

"You're bleeding?" I asked.

"No," she said. I was relieved but only momentarily. She had just learned that our dear friend Jon Barkan had died. It was a shocking and untimely death. Jon wasn't even forty years old and had a wife and three children. It made me question how I could pray for another child if God took my friend before any of his children really got to know him. I was sad, and I was angry, too. Jon helped at A Wish for Wendy and was one of those incredibly lively people who was the center of attention in any room. He was amusing, charming and a lot fun. He was also very bright and quite a leader. I used to say there were two kinds of people in this world, those who loved Jon and those who never had a chance to meet him.

Life went on, but his family and his memory would remain in my heart and mind. We had another week till we found out about our baby, but for the next few days I could only think about my friend.

As we approached shot number fourteen, the last before we found out, I prayed that this would be the final one. I was tired of putting our lives on hold to try to have a baby. I was tired of the pain Andrea was suffering. I was sick of having to wait for an answer about something so enormous. I wanted another baby, but what I didn't want was what happened on Tuesday.

Chapter 39
First Blood

Jon's funeral was on Tuesday. When his father spoke, I nearly lost it when he mentioned the children. As I listened to how Jon had taught his daughter everything he knew about sports and how they watched games and went to breakfast together, I thought of Avery and me. I thought about all of the fun we had and how that could change so quickly.

When we returned home, I took a two-hour nap. I'd been a little under the weather and needed the sleep.

At dinner, I couldn't stop crying. Having a child changed how I viewed things like this. I'd watched my friend with his daughter. I'd seen the bond between them and the fact that she would never see her father again was tearing me apart. I remembered the e-mail he sent me just weeks earlier when I asked if he could work with me again on A Wish for Wendy. Jon told me he couldn't because he had so many things he wanted to do with his kids, and I'd wished more than anything that he'd gotten that opportunity.

When I awoke from my nap, Andrea told me she'd been to the toilet and that there was blood. My heart sank. Andrea also had some spotting with Avery but this was more than normal. Still, she thought there was a decent chance that she might be pregnant. Her breasts were getting bigger, she was nauseous and she was extremely tired. All of these were good signs, but fertility doctors say there's no such thing as a good or bad sign for the first month.

That was a tough night. Andrea wanted to know what the bleeding meant and we learned on the Internet it could mean an ectopic pregnancy. That was not the kind of information we wanted to read.

Andrea fell asleep, so I had to wake her for the shot. She was too exhausted for me to rub her for the full twenty minutes so I just did fifteen, then she put on the heating pad and fell asleep again. Hopefully, I thought, that would be the worst of it.

That morning, I woke up at three o'clock to Andrea sobbing. "I don't think I'm pregnant," she cried.

The night before she seemed positive that she was. "What? Why?" I asked, but I had a feeling I knew why.

"I'm bleeding." It was Wednesday morning, just two days before we found out if we were pregnant, and Andrea started bleeding, some black and some brown, which was fine because the blood was old and could have been from her previous cycle. Some, though, was red, meaning it was fresh, and could be from her period. Every few minutes, Andrea was checking. It was driving me crazy. I couldn't sleep either. Friday could not get here quickly enough.

I hated going down early to do my therapy on Wednesday morning because Andrea wasn't awake yet. I wondered if she was still bleeding and if that would make it official that we were not pregnant. The suspense was killing me. Although we'd been told not to do it, I was beginning to think a pregnancy test might be a good idea. We had two more shots and two more mornings before we'd find out. That night we did the shot and I could tell it hurt. Andrea told me I went in too slow and I argued that I did it just like the others. It seemed each night we got a little more frustrated with the shot and, at times, each other.

We got through Thursday with little bleeding. What was there was mostly brown or black. I got the feeling Andrea was more confident, so I was getting that way, too. Still, a bad sign always seemed a moment away.

I wondered again why couldn't we just have our child and be done with it instead of having to worry about not being pregnant, or worse, an ectopic pregnancy. Why couldn't we be like our friends and have one night of fun and then a kid nine months later? It didn't seem fair, and if I sound jealous, I was.

Of course, as much as I hated IVF, I was grateful that it existed and that there were so many wonderful doctors who worked with us. Andrea and I had no chance to get pregnant without In Vitro. It was just hard while going through the process to truly appreciate it.

Thursday night, I went to sit shiva for Jon. Sitting shiva is the Jewish tradition where mourners go to a house to pray for the family and remember the person who died. I was hurting for him, but I also had tomorrow on my mind. We would finally know the result.

Friday morning was stressful. I wished Andrea a good morning as she headed to the bathroom. I didn't want to know at that point if there was more blood, so I went to feed Magic, do my therapy and lift weights. After my workout I climbed the stairs and hoped for good news. No blood. There was some hope. I thought our odds of being pregnant were about 50/50 whereas usually I put them at 30/70. We'd find out at 2:30 . . . I didn't know how I was going to be able to work.

I got home at 1:45 for the painful wait. We turned on the TV. Andrea was really worried. She was still spotting, but on the plus side, it was brown. Her breasts were still hurting and she had developed bumps on her nipples, which usually were a good sign of pregnancy. She was also quite nauseous.

Andrea asked what I thought. I told her I could not envision good news. If I did and it wasn't, I'd be devastated. I hoped for the best but I was scared. Andrea felt the same way. We'd gone back and forth for weeks. Fourteen shots, fourteen tough mornings, 384 hours since implantation, the blood, the nausea . . . we needed an answer.

At 2:35, Andrea's cell phone rang and we huddled next to it. It was Lynn, Dr. Elsner's nurse.

"Hey guys," she said. "Is Andy there?"

"Yes," I said nervously. "I'm here and I'm ready." Her voice sounded optimistic, but I didn't want to read anything into it.

"Well, you're going to be parents again!"

Andrea shouted, "Ahhhhh!" and started crying.

I was speechless. I'd been expecting the news to be bad, so I was absolutely in shock. It was four days before Wendy's birthday and we now knew that we'd again be parents. Then I thought about something else. Andrea was carrying five embryos. The chance for multiple births is quite high for fertility patients and Andrea was already starting to show at four weeks.

Every day that Andrea told me how quickly her waistline was expanding, I worried that we'd have more kids than we could handle. Andrea was more nauseous than last time and her blood levels were much higher. How many were we having?

By the time we were given a date to do the ultrasound, I was really concerned. The countdown began. When we were trying so hard to have a baby, the higher probability of having multiples seemed like a joke. Once we were pregnant, though, the joke didn't seem so funny. What if there were two? Three? Four or more? I didn't know how we'd care for all of them. We were concerned about Andrea's health, and the fact that she was thirty-four was also an issue. We didn't want to think about a reduction unless it was absolutely necessary. Andrea read that some women who had reductions had dreams about the child they removed. It was extremely difficult to think about removing one of the embryos. We had to think about Andrea's health, though, especially with everything she'd been through.

As the day got closer, Andrea and I got more and more nervous. A few nights before the ultrasound, we discussed what number we would be willing to keep. We agreed twins would be fine. We couldn't decide with triplets. We weren't sure we could handle them, but we couldn't say we'd reduce either. We decided the decision would have to be made after we knew.

I started having dreams the Sunday before the ultrasound. The first night I dreamt we had a girl, the next night twin girls, the next night one girl. Never a boy, strangely enough. Andrea's step-father joked that we were having triplets. I laughed on the outside, but on the inside I was a nervous wreck.

Then I took a moment and thought about the big picture. I shouldn't be upset; I should be happy. We got our wish! There were so many other people, even some friends, who would trade with us any day of the week and we were complaining because we might have more than one. So what? We had enough love to go around. Yes, it would be difficult. Extremely difficult, but Andrea and I had been through worse things. I was going to stop complaining. In a couple of days, we were going to hear a heartbeat—or a few heartbeats. Either way it would be wonderful.

When we got to the doctor's office, Andrea asked me what I was thinking and I told her I had so many positive thoughts and so many fears that I couldn't even say what was going through my mind. She felt the same way.

We were called to the ultrasound room and a few minutes later, our specialist came in and looked at Andrea's stomach. She said, "Wow! How many are in there?"

Now I was really freaking out. Granted, our specialist had a good sense of humor, but I was having a tough time. I paced the room while she got the machine ready. Finally, she had Andrea lie back on the chair, poured some gel on her belly and performed an ultrasound. "One heartbeat," she said.

"Really?" I said with glee.

"So far," she said.

To be honest, I'd put myself in the mind frame that I'd be happy with twins. I'd be thrilled with one . . . scared out of my mind with three. Anything more than that, I was going to have a nervous breakdown. The first time we got pregnant I'd secretly wanted twins just so we'd be done with it. I didn't want to go through the procedure again, spend all that money and deal with the emotional and physical pain.

"So, how are we looking? See any more?" I asked.

"I see a shadow," she said, "but that could just be a mirror image of the one. We'll know shortly."

I was relieved to know that worst case we had two. We could handle two. Andrea and I held hands. A few moments passed. "Well, you have just one," the specialist declared.

Andrea and I were relieved. Not that we wouldn't have loved every baby we had, but with a little girl going through the terrible twos and the time I spend on my therapy and medication, coping with multiple infants just seemed impossible. Our home would be crazy enough with two kids.

We each called our parents to let them know the good news. Andrea was seven weeks pregnant. We were going to wait to tell Avery about the baby until after her second birthday. First, it was her special day and we wanted the focus to be on her. Second, we wanted to wait until Mommy really started showing before we explained there was a baby in her stomach. Finally, we wanted to wait until we got through the first thirteen weeks of pregnancy in case we had a miscarriage.

We weren't sure if we wanted to know whether we were having a girl or boy, so we had the doctor put the information about our baby's gender in an envelope for us to open if we chose. We put it in our safe, but didn't tell our parents about the envelope because we knew they'd hound us to open it.

Andrea and I both wanted a boy. I wanted someone to continue the family name and Andrea joked that she wanted to know if a change in sex would result in the child looking more like her. We both were more concerned with the health than the gender of the baby. We thought it would be nice to have one of each, but to be honest we were truly grateful for whichever God gave us. Avery was already the best thing to ever happen to us. Anything else would be just cream on top.

Things couldn't have been better, and then, suddenly, they couldn't have been much worse.

Chapter 40
Rearing Its Ugly Head

Cystic fibrosis must take its cues from a horror movie. When the monster seems to be dead, everyone knows it's only a matter of time before it reappears stronger than ever. In January of 2008, fresh off the news that we were going to be parents again, the wrath of cystic fibrosis returned.

I was having trouble breathing and felt some extreme pressure around my chest. I tried to tell myself that it would go away, but six weeks later, the pain and breathing constriction were still there. Andrea said I should call the doctor, but I dreaded making that call more than anything. Normally I'm pretty tough when it comes to facing medical issues, but I'd never been so afraid to see Dr. Stecenko.

I had a daughter now. Andrea was pregnant, nauseous all the time, and couldn't help as she normally did. I was afraid of the seriousness of an infection. Would I have to be hospitalized? Would I die before my baby was born? Would I be helpless when my children needed me? These questions created a level of fear I'd never experienced. My prior staph infections were scary only because I was worried about me. This was about my children and my wife, and to me they were far more important. I couldn't help thinking of my friend who had just died and left a wife and three children.

My depression grew. Fear raced through my mind. I played about fifty games of pool over the next two days. Striking the pool balls temporarily relieved my frustration. My mother came and gave me a pep talk, telling me I would be fine and to smile more.

"Come on, Andy," she demanded. "Snap out of it!"

The more she said it, the more aggravated I grew.

"Where's the Andy I know?" she asked.

My father, ever the problem solver, called me from a business trip in New York. He asked what the issue was and insisted that whatever it was, "we'd take care of it." The problem was, we didn't know what the problem was. I couldn't be the positive Andy until I knew what I was up against.

Everyone was irritating me. Andrea tried to be strong, but she was hormonal, and in her eyes I could see the hurt and fear of losing her husband and taking care of two kids by herself.

On a Tuesday, I went for a chest X-ray. I was frustrated that I couldn't get my PFTs that day because the Emory Clinic was booked. The following day I went for my pulmonary function test and a visit with Dr. Stecenko. I tried to tell myself that maybe it wasn't as bad as I thought. After all, my oxygen levels and weight were normal. After the PFTs, Andrea and I waited for the doctor. Usually I came by myself but this time I needed moral support. I'd been depressed over the last twenty-four hours because Dr. Stecenko thought I could have pneumonia or pleurisy.

"So your PFTs are down," Dr. Stecenko said.

"Way down?" I asked, hoping to somehow pull good news out of bad.

"Yes," she said.

I freaked out. Was it thirty percent like several years ago? She told me it was only seven percent, so I calmed down a bit. I'd also just caught a cold, so I blamed half of the seven percent on that, but I had grown three bacteria. Staph, as usual, was one of the culprits. I had a serious infection in the lower left lobe so she added two new meds to my mix. I was instructed to use my vest twice a day, inhale a twenty-minute mist three times a day, and report back in three weeks. Every afternoon around lunch, I left my office, ducked into my car, drove to an abandoned parking lot and did my second mist of the day.

During those three weeks, I tried to find a positive spin. My numbers were not staggeringly lower than normal and I still had enough energy to work out and help with Avery. The doctor said my chest sounded pretty clear and I wasn't losing any weight. Sure, I was going to have to take a lot more meds and do therapy for nearly two hours a day, but I knew things were going to get better.

I started making a list of what I could do to get well. I was going to do a lot more running and get back into tennis. I'd taken some time off, but we owned a tennis ball machine that would be good for more exercise. I would start using my push up grips. I'd start walking the dog around the cul-de-sac every night. I set a date for being back to 100 percent. It was the same day as the start of Andrea's third trimester.

I wasn't going down without a fight. Mr. Positive was back.

Unfortunately, while my mind was positive, my results weren't. Three weeks later, not only had I not improved, my PFTs were down another 10 percent. I guess I already knew it. As positive as I tried to be, I was still out of breath from minimal athletic activity and I could feel the obstruction in my airways. It was frustrating, doing five therapies a day, taking three different antibiotics, exercising hard in the gym, yet still getting negative results. It was time to face facts. For the first time in my life, I needed to go on IV antibiotics.

Dr. Stecenko was surprised I'd gone so long without them. Most cystic fibrosis patients endured IV antibiotics multiple times during their lives. She told me I would be okay. Her confidence was reassuring. Dr. Boat also called to tell me he agreed with Dr. Stecenko's strategy. Because he has known me for so long, he knew I would want his input.

Thankfully, I was able to have the IV at home with a nurse, but it would still be inconvenient. I told myself if this was what it took to get better then this was what I had to do. The problem was that Avery's second birthday was that Saturday. I didn't want to miss it, so we made the initial appointment—which had to be at the clinic—for one o'clock the following Monday, several hours after Andrea's thirteen week ultrasound.

Avery's party was terrific. Only my close friends knew that I was sick, as I wanted the party to be about Avery and not her dad. Two days later, we headed to the ultrasound. The baby looked great in the ultrasound pictures and the heartbeat sounded strong. We went for hibachi and then to the radiology department at the Emory Clinic to have the PICC line for the IV inserted.

The doctor had me lie on a bed with my arm positioned on a perpendicular board. The doctor injected medicine to numb the pain, then proceeded to lace a noodle-like string in my arm and attached the line to it. The procedure was painful and took about twenty-five minutes. Afterward a home care service nurse named Stuart met us at the house. As we got out of the car, I noticed my arm was bleeding. I freaked out, but Stuart said it was relatively normal, and quickly cleaned it.

Over the next few hours he showed us how to administer the medication. It was a little frightening how precise every little thing had to be. For example, just to administer one of the four daily meds, I had to lay out all my supplies (alcohol wipe, saline flush, antibiotic), sterilize the PICC line with alcohol, open the PICC line clamp and inject saline to flush the line, sterilize the line again, then open the bag of antibiotic solution and connect it with the line. The hardest part was making sure everything remained absolutely clean and that I didn't touch any foreign objects during the procedure.

Stuart warned me that one little mistake could land me in the hospital with a serious infection. I had to administer the drug Zosyn three times daily in twenty minute intervals and the drug Tobramycin once a day for an hour. That was another two hours added to the two and a half hours I was already spending with aerosol and vest therapies. I had to take a pill before any of the IVs, so my first treatment started at five-thirty in the morning and my last treatment of the day ended around eleven at night.

The second day, Stuart removed the tape and wiped the area with alcohol to remove the blood. The procedure was painful, but necessary. The following day, he took three vials of blood and continued to monitor my condition. I had trouble going upstairs to see Avery or Andrea. I did not even have the stamina to read a children's book to Avery. I was out of breath and exhausted. I just hated that I wasn't myself.

The basement went from being "the man room" to a dungeon. I was sick of sitting in there. I couldn't work out, play pool or go outside to shoot hoops. My stomach hurt from the IVs and I had constant diarrhea. I could not lift anything above six pounds and, of course, that meant not being able to hold my precious Avery. I even had difficulty opening the caps on some of my meds and had trouble flushing the line with saline. I freaked out quite often. Even with the smallest hiccup, I would scream at the top of my lungs for Andrea to help me. I wasn't just physically struggling. Despite my earlier positive attitude, I was depressed. My friends were very supportive and several of them brought dinner the first week I was on IVs, or dropped by to cheer me up. A neighbor, whose sons played with Avery, offered to take her whenever we needed a break. Co-workers offered to help with whatever we needed and my parents were there almost every night. It was comforting to know we had all of these people to help us. It made me realize that if something happened to me, they would take care of Andrea and Avery. I smiled and told everyone I could beat this and that they shouldn't be too concerned.

The truth was, I was terrified.

Chapter 41
Struggling to Find Strength

Having friends visit was nice, but as soon as they left the depression returned. I felt bad for Andrea, who had to do most of the work. She was pregnant, working a full-time job, taking care of a two-year-old, and worrying about her ailing husband.

I wanted to wake up and magically be well, but as each day passed, it was apparent that would not happen. Softball season was only a month away and I wasn't in shape to play. I'd already taken my name off the tennis team roster. I started thinking about the Peachtree Road Race, which was just five months away. My streak was now in jeopardy.

After a week, the PICC line began to itch and dry blood had spread around the region. Stuart came back the following Monday to clean it. He took my vital signs and told me that my blood pressure was high. "Duh," I thought, "I'm just a little stressed here." I fell asleep after Stuart left and when I woke up I slowly pulled myself out of bed and walked upstairs. Mom and Dad were there along with Andrea and Avery and Mom tried to cheer me up. I felt like I was part of some sort of intervention.

"Andy," she begged, "go outside. Get out of here for a while."

I refused. I felt like a hermit living a miserable life underground who only emerged for an occasional meal or to sit on the couch. I went to the bathroom and looked at myself in the mirror. I had a beard growing out of control, a rash that spread from my forearm to just below my shoulder and a constant frown on my face. A torn sock covered my PICC line. My hair was a mess. My forehead was breaking out from the antibiotics and I hadn't bathed in several days. Prior to administrating the IVs, I was up at 5:30 to work out and do my therapy. Now I was lucky if I woke up at eleven. Every time I looked at my reflection, I grew more depressed.

Mom looked at Andrea and said, "He always was like that. He hates to talk. When he was younger, he would do the same thing. He would not talk to us, but then he would go outside and play sports and feel better."

Andrea begged me, "Go outside and take a drive." My mom kept bugging me about snapping out of my depression. Her nagging finally touched

199

a nerve. Maybe it was thinking about being eight years old again. Maybe I remembered my old babysitter or the awkward circumstance with the family friend. I was in bad shape then, but had been inspired by the poster of a bigger-than-life man who showed me I could live a long life. I'd gotten so close to being as muscular as that guy, and now I'd regressed to that eight-year-old child fighting for every breath. But the truth was that I wasn't fighting. I was giving in.

I grabbed the car keys and muttered that I needed to take a drive. In the car I turned up the music as loud as I could, opened the sunroof and drove straight to the tennis courts. As I watched two men playing, my eyes welled with tears. I didn't really see the players—I saw me.

"You can do it!" I shouted as I beat my fists on the steering wheel. "Don't give up!"

I looked in the mirror, and despite the beard and long hair I saw a glimpse of the old me. I saw him begging to come out. I knew then I was going to renew my efforts and fight this thing with everything I had. That night, I wrote a letter to my friends.

Dear Friends:

I want to thank all of you for your calls, e-mails and meals. It means a lot. If I don't call you back, please don't take it the wrong way. I just have good days and bad. I've been strapped to the IV for more than a week now, going through five-hour treatments. I'm exhausted by the ordeal and dealing with the pain of giving blood every few days. I feel like a pin cushion lately. To be quite honest, I've been depressed, too.

Andrea has been so helpful and so supportive and my parents have helped, too. Last night was a breakthrough for me. I drove around alone and in that isolation I was finally able to break down. Sometimes you need to explode and let it all out to find what's missing. Lately, I've used all my energy in a negative way, worrying about the future instead of focusing on making the future better.

It's time for me to take my future to a new level. I now look forward to beating cystic fibrosis. It may not be a week or two weeks, but in the end, I will win. I have set a goal to be 100 percent by the time baby number two arrives.

Today begins my comeback; thanks again for your constant support.

I've been knocked down, but now I'm ready to get back up.

Andy

The following day I got my own lunch instead of waiting for Andrea or my mom to bring it to me. On Wednesday, I took Magic for a two-mile walk. I even ran a mile of it, and I felt a little better. I was not as out of breath as I expected to be, and would have gone out again if it hadn't been thirty degrees outside.

Things were starting to look up. I had a doctor's appointment on Friday. I was prepared for bad news, but worked to make the news better. Avery had gymnastics class that day, so an unlikely candidate volunteered to take me to the doctor: my mother. Mom hadn't been to the doctor with me in nearly two decades. I'd blown up at her then, but promised myself that no matter the outcome, this time I wouldn't get upset. Mom talked the entire trip, but that didn't distract me from the pending visit with my doctor. What if I still wasn't better?

On my first attempted blow on my PFT, I coughed and had to start over. The nurse gave me some water and I tried again. This time I gave a full blow. I thought I nailed it, but the nurse revealed it was even lower than last time. I tried again and again without improvement. I wondered if the IV antibiotics were a waste of time. I got on the phone with Dr. Stecenko and she told me she was having the PICC line removed and that I'd need another chest X-ray. After reviewing it, she called to say there was very little difference from the last one. The next step was a CT scan.

My father called to say that he would call Dr. Boat at home to see what he thought. I didn't want to talk about it anymore. My positive attitude had eroded along with my PFT scores, and I felt that whenever I spoke to my father, the conversation was only about my health. In fact, I didn't want to talk to either of my parents because—like well-meaning, loving parents sometimes do—they drove me crazy. Emily thought I should go see Dr. Boat. I just wanted a break.

A few nights after my last conversation with Dr. Stecenko, Andrea had had it with me. "Where is your fight, Andy? I've tried to be supportive, but you're not trying. I've never seen you like this. I thought when you sent the e-mail to your friends that you'd gotten over the hump, but now you're back where you started. Do it for your daughter. She loves you so much."

As if she knew it were her cue, Avery scurried up and hugged my leg, not once but twice. It was an emotional and humbling moment, but I knew what I had to do. I had to dig deep and fight this so my daughter had a father. I owed it to her. I owed it to our next baby, and to my wife. I owed it to myself.

The problem was that as much as I wanted to be an inspiration to my loved ones, I could not find the energy. I could not get out of this rut. I felt I was a royal disappointment to everyone. It was as if my self-esteem levels as a child and college student had returned, or my biggest fear... they'd never left. Still, I knew I could not flinch. I had to pull myself together. With renewed determination I spoke to Dr. Boat and he told me to have the CT scan sent to him as soon as it was done. Dr. Stecenko was out of town, but she put the head adult pulmonologist in charge of my care while she was away. That is how I was introduced to Dr. Wolfenden.

I took the tennis ball machine and forty-eight balls to our neighborhood courts and hit the full batch four times. My goal was that not a single ball would bounce twice even though I had the machine moving the ball from one side to the other. At the end, I ran suicide sprints, touching every line on the tennis court and darting back to the fence after each touch. I was exhausted, but I knew the only way to start getting better was to get out and get my mind off the situation. As I drove home, I saw Andrea walking toward me with Avery and Magic. They had come to surprise me and to show how proud they were of me for getting back out there.

As luck would have it, instead of things getting better, they only got worse. Avery woke up vomiting during the night. The following day, Andrea caught the same virus. I was at work for the first time in two weeks when Andrea called me to tell me she was sick. As I sat in my office, I too, began to feel cold and nauseous. I went home and lay next to Andrea with a 102-degree fever, a bad headache, and a feeling that Murphy's Law would soon be changed to Lipman's Law. Two days later, it was my father's turn to take me to the doctor. Dr. Wolfenden looked at my CT scan and said it didn't look too bad, but there were definite places of infection. My PFTs had not changed and she thought I needed another round of IV antibiotics. That frustrated me, since I'd only had the PICC line removed a week earlier. Dr. Boat concurred with Dr. Wolfenden's decision and I decided to use her as my primary Atlanta physician, since she'd dealt with more adults with CF than Dr. Stecenko.

After a three-hour wait due to a miscommunication, another PICC line was placed in my arm. The doctor tried to put the line in my left arm so I could play sports, but she hit a nerve and I cried out. After forty minutes of trying, she gave up. My left arm had a bruise six inches long. At this point, I was in pain and had the chills. Thirty minutes later, the PICC line was inserted in my right arm and I went home to sleep.

The next morning, I learned that to get the medication I needed, I had to see an infectious disease doctor, who would monitor me. Andrea was furious and called the doctor to argue that the meds needed to be started immediately and that the CF Center could check my vitals. She didn't want me to drive, then wait several more hours just to get the okay to take some drugs. Thanks to Andrea, I got the medicine that night. I'd be taking a drug called Vancomycin once in the morning and once at night. Each session would take eighty minutes.

Since the IV was in my right arm, I made a decision to become left-handed. I went to hit tennis balls with my Aunt Susie for an hour. It was like starting over again, but two days after starting my meds, I was a hitting a little bit better off the ball machine and was not as out of breath. A few days later, I was hitting the ball like I did right-handed. I didn't have the aim yet, but I was hitting some great shots. I began to love the challenge of becoming ambidextrous.

Later that week, Dr. Wolfenden called with the results of my latest sputum culture and blood test. My kidney function had gone down quite a bit so she took me off the Tobramycin, which is known to contribute to poor kidney function. The sputum culture revealed I had acquired MRSA, a strong staph bug. The good news was that the Vancomycin I was taking would help with the MRSA. The bad news is that I would later find out that I was allergic to Vancomycin. The drug caused a rash to develop on each of my arms which caused a severe itch.

When I went back in to see Dr. Wolfenden two weeks later, my numbers had gone up five percent. I was ecstatic. Things were finally moving in the right direction. She wanted to start me on another antibiotic, Zyvox, one I'd tried orally several years before that gave me a rash on my testicles. It was pretty awful then, but she said if I took it with Benadryl and because it would be an IV, the problem was less likely. When she pointed out that studies showed it was more effective against MRSA than what I was currently getting, I knew I had to take the risk. How else could I get better?

Zyvox had to be given through a bag suspended from an IV pole. I was a little intimidated by having to pop the bag and hang it on the pole so the medicine would dispense properly. Andrea agreed to set it up every day before work and every night before my last dose. She was a real trooper through the entire process. I feared that I was putting a lot of strain on her, but the only thing that scared me more was screwing up the proper way to administer the medication and having to be admitted to a hospital. I had to have two doses, each lasting two hours. The other transition I had to make was that the IV pole was far less portable than the pressure-filled containers I'd used previously.

I started feeling better and a week after I began the new round of medication, I was playing tennis left-handed with ease. I was also able to work out more regularly. Just maybe, life was getting better.

Then, on a Friday, I took a bath. It was difficult to take a shower because the PICC line could slip out of my arm if I got it wet. So, holding my arm over the edge of the bathtub was far less risky, especially since Andrea wrapped my arm in plastic. In the tub, I noticed my right testicle had a pink spot on it. It didn't itch nor hurt, but I thought it could be the rash coming back. That Saturday, it began to hurt and got progressively worse. It was like a serious form of jock itch. The entire area turned pink with dark red bumps, and by Sunday, I could hardly walk. The pain was excruciating. I called Emory's after-hours line and was surprised when Dr. Caplan answered. It was a little awkward because we hadn't talked in the two decades since I'd left his practice. He asked how I was and how my parents were, but since he was the only doctor on call, he kept the small talk to a minimum. He prescribed some medicated powder, but it did little good. Andrea suggested I just stop taking the drug, but I only had four days left and I couldn't stop now. I used some Lotrimin on the rash and felt slightly better.

My next set of PFTs showed no change. Another disappointment. I was visibly upset. Dr. Wolfenden looked from me to Andrea, then back at me. "Don't let one piece of paper determine if you'll get better," she said. That line has stuck with me ever since.

I nodded, knowing that it was great advice, but when she left to set up my next appointment, I began crying. I had worked so hard and the tests proved there was nothing to show for it.

"It's okay," said Andrea, her own eyes welling up. "Maybe you should accept the fact that as you get older your lung function won't be as good as you want it. We all get worse off with age, whether we have CF or not."

As I listened to her, I realized the warrior in me wasn't done. I refused to accept that I wouldn't get better, refused to ask less of myself, refused to give up and refused to accept. I wanted to be the exception.

We tried to hug, but I stopped the embrace to say, "Don't give up on me, Sweetie. I will get better. I won't let this beat me." That was the old me, the one who was missing for so long during the IV antibiotics.

That evening I sent an update to my friends:

> Dear Family and Friends,
>
> Well, I went to the doctor and there's good news and not so good news. The good news is that my sinuses looked pretty clear and I was able to have the PICC line removed. This means in twenty-four hours I can use both my arms to hug my wife and daughter. The bad news is that my lung function did not improve, but it didn't go down either, so I can go back to my full workouts, and softball; and the rash should be going away soon. They took several vials of blood (sixteen in fact) and will do some gastro studies. The doctor isn't too concerned. She said that compared to most with CF, I'm doing well and that we will get to the bottom of this. Unfortunately, she would not validate our parking but it was worth a shot. I don't know about shaving the beard, but I probably will since I'm going to be working out a lot more. I'll be heading back to the office for some "normalcy" on Monday or Tuesday.

Some have asked if I feel unfortunate. Sure. I'd be lying if I said I didn't, but my overwhelming feeling is that I have a chance to prove to myself and everyone around me what kind of fighter I am. I'm not going down. I'm going to hire a personal trainer, get back into running, and working out with heavier weights. I also plan to hit .600 this season and I don't plan to use a pinch runner. I'm going to prove to cystic fibrosis that it picked the wrong person when it picked me. Cystic fibrosis is the one with a fight on its hands.

Thank you to everyone for the kind words, the prayers and everything else. I do intend to beat this. I will get better.

Never take a day for granted.

Andy

With the IV removed, I intended to go back to my normal activities and add the personal trainer to the list; that is until we got the call from my Aunt Anita. I was devastated to learn that Uncle Jerry had succumbed to brain cancer. He was only fifty-eight.

When Andrea and I arrived in Charleston for the funeral, Aunt Anita told me that the two of them had thought about me a lot over the past few months. I also learned that my uncle told my mother just before he died that he worried about me and that he would pray for me. It was hard for me to imagine that a man on his death bed was praying for me, but that's the kind of guy Uncle Jerry was.

It was he and my Aunt Anita who brought Howard to me when I was little. The fondest memory I have of my uncle is when I was in Charleston and my therapy machine broke. I had no way of doing my therapy other than having Andrea do the old fashioned chest thumping method of postural drainage. But my uncle wouldn't hear of it. On a Saturday he called some contacts, reached a man who worked at the small company that made my machine and arranged to have a new one delivered by nightfall. Uncle Jerry helped me out that day. I only wished I could have done the same for him. I thought I should dedicate my comeback to him. And I did.

As soon as we got home I shaved most of my beard, leaving only a goatee. I started playing tennis, working out and playing softball again. In my first game I went 1-for-3 with an RBI and a nice catch in the outfield. I hired a personal trainer, David Caplan (no relation to Dr. Caplan), to work with me every Tuesday and Thursday for ten weeks and, through him, I began to improve my nutrition and diet. The workouts were difficult, but I tried as hard as I could to do them, just like everyone else. Unlike everyone else, I did more than David asked of me. I told him I would be his hardest working client and I meant it. Between sessions with the trainer, I continued my own exercise routine. I felt like I was in Coach Mervos' class again.

After missing two months of work, I went back into the office where I got hugs, handshakes and questions about why I was donning facial hair.

Having both arms to play sports and being able to shower again were great, but the best thing about getting the PICC line removed was holding Avery and Andrea. I really missed that. I told Avery every time she hugged me that each hug had to be the best one ever and she always complied. I was able to play games with her, put her to bed and take more of a role in her life.

One day I took Avery to a carnival. Now able to use both arms, I wanted to try the basketball shooting game. The man working the booth told my father only one guy had won all weekend because the hoop was the same size as the ball and the rim had no give to it. I missed my first three shots, but decided to try four more. On my final try the ball hit the rim, bounced five times, and swished into the bottom of the net. I won a huge stuffed dog for Avery, who must have hugged it at least twenty times that afternoon. Winning was another boost to my confidence and proof once again that the most unlikely results really can happen. I'd learned that lesson many times, but it never hurt to get a reminder.

Chapter 42
The Enigma

Over the next few months, things were getting better for me. Doctor Wolfenden had informed me that my PFT numbers were up four percent. Her exact words were, "Andy, this is awesome! I'm thrilled with these numbers." It seemed that I'd finally gotten my health under control.

I'd caught my first foul ball in my thirty-plus years of attending baseball games. I framed the ball, my ticket, the game program and the box score in a 12" x 12" wooden frame and hung it in my basement. It had always been a dream of mine to catch a foul ball.

With my health improving, I no longer worried about IV antibiotics or any antibiotics for that matter. That summer, I was even able to continue my streak and run another Peachtree Road Race. I finished it in just over an hour beating my prior year's time by more than five minutes.

I'd also gotten to take the trip of a lifetime with my close friend Ross Jacobs in May of that year. Andrea had surprised me with two tickets to the two stadiums I most wanted to see—Yankee Stadium in New York and Fenway Park in Boston. I was a big fan of baseball history and always wanted to see the stadiums where baseball greats Babe Ruth, Ted Williams and Lou Gehrig once played. She paid for our limo ride to the airport, our airfare, our hotels and our tickets. She even packed my bags before I got home for the surprise. She knew it would mean a lot to go with Ross. He lived with me for four years and helped me get through some of my toughest times with CF. He was my best man at my wedding and I was his. To this day, that surprise trip is the coolest thing anyone has ever done for me.

Still the excitement was only just beginning.

I couldn't believe it. August was finally here. I'd counted down the days for the last two months. My parents had a trip to Israel planned so they wanted to know if they should be back for a bris, so that July we decided to find out what we were having. As they say at the Oscars, the envelope please. We were expecting a boy . . . the family name would be kept intact. Avery would have a baby brother, and I would have a son to escort to Little League games. I felt the birth of my son was going to change my luck. In fact, my luck had already begun to change. At my most recent doctor's appointment, I'd learned my lung function showed a whopping 12 percent improvement. I was at my baseline lung function just in time for the birth of our baby boy.

Andrea's mom and step-dad came into town the Saturday before the scheduled birth to help us prepare for the baby's arrival. It was a busy weekend. We took Avery to two birthday parties. Everyone asked about Andrea and what was going through my head with the new arrival only hours away. I was thrilled because one of the things that motivated me to get better was the birth of my son.

On August 12th, Andrea and I were due at the hospital at six in the morning for a C-section. Andrea didn't want a Caesarian, but her doctor thought it best because she'd already had one. I couldn't sleep that night. So, around 1:30 I headed down to do my therapy. I heard footsteps running down the stairs, which was unusual at that time of the morning. I figured it was Andrea wondering why I was up so early. It was Andrea, but that's not why she was up. She opened the basement door, hustled down the stairs and told me she had fluid running down her leg and the baby wasn't moving. Suddenly she could run and stretch when she hadn't been able to the last three months.

By three o'clock we were heading to Piedmont Hospital in a panic. The nurse, who happened to be the same one we had when Avery was born, immediately found our son's heartbeat on the monitor and said he was fine. It wasn't much reassurance. I hoped the poor start to the day was not an omen.

Shortly thereafter, Andrea delivered our second child, a baby boy we named Ethan Cole after our grandfathers, Erwin and Carl. I thought about one of Ethan's Hebrew names, Nissim, which means miracle. We named him that because going through successful IVF to have a child was truly a miracle. I was going to call Ethan "E" and tell everyone that if my grandfather met Ethan he would have said, "E, I'm Carl." If you scramble the letters in that sentence, it reads "miracle." Ethan's other Hebrew name was Zacharia, meaning "in memory," which was after Wendy.

Ethan, who was not quite the spitting image of me that Avery was, had blonde hair and blue eyes and was eight pounds ten ounces at birth. He looked like a healthy baby, but, after taking a lot of pictures, I got the impression something was wrong. Really wrong!

"Please don't take any more pictures," one of the nurses said as we were walking from the operating room to the nursery. I didn't remember the nurse telling me that when Avery was born. This nurse wanted to rush Ethan into the nursery.

"His oxygen levels are a little low," I heard another nurse say. They also noted his breathing was very heavy.

"Oh, God," I thought. "What's wrong with my son?"

Terrible thoughts crept into my mind. Could he have CF? Would I have to leave my own son when he had an infection? Andrea was tested for the cystic fibrosis gene, but there are some gene mutations that cannot be detected, so even if the test was negative, there was still a chance the child could have CF. Ethan was being examined by the doctors in the nursery, and I had to face my wife who had just gotten out of major surgery and pretend Ethan was fine.

"What's wrong?" Andrea asked.

"Nothing, I'm just tired," I replied. I knew she could read me, and part of me wanted her to so I didn't have to shock her with the news that our son was sick. I went from Andrea's room to the nursery five times hoping for good news, but each time Ethan seemed to have more wires connected to him. What were they looking for, I wondered?

I grew frustrated, especially as other babies left the nursery to join their parents. Later that afternoon I met with Dr. Weil, the pediatrician on call.

"Looks like some fluid in the lungs, most likely from the C-section." The tall doctor, who donned a dark beard and mustache, said he would probably be fine. I had prepared for much worse.

Ethan was moved to the intermediate care nursery, a bridge nursery between the regular nursery and the NICU (Neonatal Intensive Care Unit). No one wanted their child in the NICU. Dr. Weil said Ethan was there as a precaution so they could monitor his breathing. None of the doctors seemed too concerned.

I still had doubts, but reluctantly decided to send the announcement that Ethan was born and that a bris was planned a week later. In the next few hours, I received nearly fifty congratulatory e-mails and phone calls, and several confirmations from people who would be attending the bris. I told myself I was worried about nothing. The fact that people were booking flights to come to see Ethan should be the least of my concerns.

Andrea insisted I spend the first night at home, since Ethan would be staying in the nursery all night. She was devastated that she was not able to hold her baby until that evening. He still couldn't be brought to our room due to concerns about how he would adapt to the temperature change. The nurses needed to monitor him and the doctors were concerned he might be susceptible to germs. Hearing babies on either side of our room joining their parents for bonding time was extremely difficult. Andrea and I were stuck watching the Beijing Olympics and staring at each other.

Andrea was allowed to breast feed Ethan that evening. My wife is a firm believer in breastfeeding. Nothing would stop her. She breastfed Avery for over a year and that night she fed Ethan four times. I was so proud of her. She could have taken that time to sleep and recover, but instead she asked the nurses to wake her and wheel her to the nursery so she could feed our child.

When Andrea and I spoke the following morning she said Ethan looked better, but I needed to hear it from the doctors, so I called the nursery at six-thirty in the morning.

"How's Ethan?" I asked.

"He's okay," the nurse said. Her tone concerned me.

"Okay," I said. "Anything wrong?"

"Ethan had some saturation issues this morning," she said. "His SAT rate went from 100 percent to under eighty." Apparently the saturation rate determined how well Ethan was taking in oxygen.

I called Andrea who was unaware of the problem. She made some inquiries, then called to tell me the doctor wanted to do tests and to hurry in so she wouldn't be alone for the news. I called my parents and they hurried to join us.

Ethan's SAT rates went down again later that day. I was there when it happened. He started turning blue, a loud monitor went off, and the nurses began giving him oxygen and gently moving him so he would breathe again. I was in shock. What was wrong with our son? What was happening to him?

Dr. Parellada, the pediatrician on call, had Ethan moved to the NICU for further tests. He wanted to do an MRI and an EEG. He told us this was normal procedure and that he'd let us know the results. It seemed like our lives were spent waiting for results, but waiting to find out what was happening to our little boy was one of the hardest things I have ever experienced.

Andrea's father, Manny, came that night and Andrea cried on his shoulder. She and her dad went to feed Ethan around eleven. I'd fallen asleep watching the Olympics but at eleven-fifteen I awoke to a nightmare.

Manny ran in and shook me, "Ethan had a seizure. Andrea is with him. Let's go."

I jumped up and threw on my running shoes, not caring that I still wore my blue pajamas. I ran to the NICU two hallways down and found Andrea with her hands covering her head. I could hear her crying fifty feet away. I thought Ethan had died. I looked over to see him lying with a tube and wires attached to him. My heart, which had been thumping mightily, nearly stopped when I saw he was still breathing.

Andrea was hysterical. Ethan had a seizure while Andrea was feeding him and the nurses were quite sure the same thing had happened before. Our hearts sank when we heard Ethan's SAT rate had gone from one hundred to under twenty, which basically is not breathing. We left so they could do more tests.

"Seizures!" sobbed Andrea. "Do you know what that means, Andy? Why us?"

I tried to act strong but I wondered the same thing. Why us? Why always us? We spent a long, grueling night wondering, watching, and waiting.

Dr. Parellada came the following morning to say most of Ethan's tests were normal but they were still waiting on the MRI. That was good news. I could tell Andrea was becoming more optimistic too. Maybe this was a freak thing. Maybe the seizure was a false diagnosis. But moments later we had a call from Dr. Parellada. Ethan's EEG indicated he had been having active seizures yesterday. I clenched my teeth, trying to stop the tears. I grabbed Andrea to hug her, but Andrea didn't have time for hugs. She called a co-worker at the CDC, an emergency room doctor named Jerry Thomas. We had talked the night before, just after Ethan's seizure, but we needed him there, in person. He arrived later that morning to translate Ethan's results and explain what the doctors were really saying. I don't know what we would have done without him.

Ethan had had an infarct, which was a stroke that occurred in his brain, and Dr. Parellada believed a significant portion of the brain was affected. He showed us the MRI, which Jerry helped us translate. Dr. Parellada didn't sound optimistic. I left Andrea with her father so they could talk and went with my mom to pick up food. For the first time I was able to have a good cry. I felt like a child again, crying on my mother's shoulder. "Why Ethan?" I sobbed. I told my mother that I now understood some of what they went through with me and with Wendy. My mother held me and told me I had to stay positive. We would get through this. That afternoon, I cancelled Ethan's bris.

I tried to remain calm and confident because I knew I had to be there for Andrea. I thought about my parents and what must be going through their minds, re-living a nightmare of nearly four decades ago. Andrea's father told me that my dad called this "the toughest day" of his life. It reminded him so much of Wendy, and he didn't want me to have to go through that. My parents were at the hospital around the clock to check on Ethan and talk with the doctors.

We decided to transfer Ethan to Scottish Rite Children's Hospital, because it had child neurology specialists who could help. Andrea and I were shocked when, before leaving for Scottish Rite, the delivery team brought Ethan to us in a contraption that looked like a space-aged aquarium.

It was the first time Ethan had been in our hospital room and it had been almost seventy-two hours since his birth. Andrea and I cried, but with tears of happiness, as we sensed these people would help Ethan. They told us how cute he was and that he was going to get better. My father was the sole rider in the ambulance with Ethan going to Scottish Rite. That evening, Dr. Howard Schub, a neurologist at Scottish Rite and friend of my parents, called to tell us he'd examined Ethan and was encouraged that he seemed to have full control of all of his extremities. He was put on phenobarbital to control the seizures, but the doctors weren't sure it would be effective.

I was with Andrea, who could not be released from Piedmont until the following day due to their surgical protocol. She got a release for the evening so that we could go and feed Ethan. Both of my parents were at Scottish Rite when we arrived. The children's hospital was very uplifting with pretty colors on all the walls. There was an enormous fish tank at the entrance and the elevators were named after beautiful outdoorsy things like flowers and butterflies. Here, each nurse was assigned only two children. A two-to-one ratio was much better than the five-to-one at Piedmont. A doctor was assigned to get Ethan's information from Piedmont, and she followed up on Ethan's expanded genetic screening, which had been sent to the lab shortly after he was born. The doctor also took our family's medical history and reviewed all of Ethan's tests.

After Andrea fed Ethan and we had some quality time to spend with our son, we reluctantly left so that I could bring Andrea back to the hospital.

Each time my cell phone rang on the ride home after dropping off Andrea at Piedmont, I worried that it was Dr. Schub calling to say that Ethan's condition worsened and that I'd have to share the news with Andrea. During Ethan's first few days on earth, it seemed every time I sat down, the phone rang with bad news about our son. I arrived home to spend some time with Avery who was with Andrea's mom and stepfather. She had no idea what was going on and that's how I tried to keep it. Prior to Ethan's birth, I envisioned taking her to Piedmont to visit her brother, but I knew now that this was impossible. Andrea had even bought Avery a blue dress that read "Ethan's Big Sister" that she planned for her to wear when she met Ethan at the hospital.

In my heart, I felt dead. I had gone through so much that my entire being was numb. At home I didn't sleep. I just put my head on the pillow and stared uncomprehendingly at the TV. When people talked to me, their words had no meaning. I called my friends and they allowed me to talk and cry while they listened. I understand now that for a parent, having a sick child is like living in the depths of darkness.

The next morning, as Andrea's father and I left the hospital for the final time, Dr. Parellada stopped us. He said he hoped Ethan got better and was surprised how great he looked. I know he meant that he was amazed how good Ethan looked, despite the seizures.

"Your son is an enigma," he said.

I didn't say it aloud, but I thought to myself, "He's not an enigma. He's a Lipman. We prove doctors wrong. You'll see."

The tests continued to come back normal and Ethan had not had additional episodes. Exactly one week after his birth, we were cleared to take our son home. We would have to keep him on a monitor for his breathing and continue to give him phenobarbital twice daily. We also hired a night nurse for the first month; it was a small price to pay to have our son home. Andrea and I were ecstatic to pick up Ethan and host a family gathering to welcome him home. A very excited Avery finally got to wear her "Ethan's Big Sister" dress and couldn't quit grinning at him. Slowly, I was able to envision having a Little Leaguer again.

The bris was held a few weeks later. Rabbi Joshua Heller, who visited Ethan while at Scottish Rite, reminded us of the Hebrew name we gave him. I thought about the word "miracle," which Nissim signified.

Rabbi Heller said it best. "Sometimes we pick a name out for a person . . . and sometimes a name just picks out a person."

Ethan was our little miracle—in more ways than one.

Chapter 43
Not Afraid to Tri!

By the following summer, things seemed to be back on track. Ethan was nearly a year old, the doctors were happy with his progress, and he was finally off the apnea monitor he'd been on since we brought him home.

That June, Andrea and I attempted our first triathlons. I was never a good swimmer. In fact, I remembered being six or seven years old when Josh and other friends competed in CF swimming fundraisers at the Fontainebleau Swimming Club while I watched. I couldn't take part because CF inhibited my ability to hold my breath underwater, so I sat on the sidelines feeling alienated. That flashback motivated me. I took lessons for a month at a swimming facility near work to get good enough to even practice for a triathlon. The swim required going a distance of sixteen lengths in an Olympic-sized pool. I joined a gym with a pool and swam once or twice a week. I started at one length and a month later was at five lengths. Soon I was able to do the sixteen lengths. Eventually I got up to twenty.

I e-mailed Aaron Spitalnick, a friend I hadn't seen in more than a decade, to borrow his bike. It was great to see him when I went to pick up the bike and especially to see how much his daughter meant to him. He still threw a few social and CF jabs my way like it was old times, but it was obvious how much he had matured and how much his daughter changed his life.

I trained only a few days for the twelve-mile bike ride. The run was a five-kilometer race, which, due to my Peachtree practice, would be the easiest of the three legs. Even with all my practice for the swim, it was much more difficult than I imagined. First, the venue wasn't a pool, but rather a lake where I could not touch the bottom. Secondly, there were 800 other people kicking and swiping at me while we swam the quarter mile. Third, I didn't weigh 180 pounds anymore. Ethan's spell in the hospital and my time on IVs had ignited my depression. As my depression worsened, I ate more and gained weight despite working out, which was ironic since CF patients are known for being skinny. I weighed just over 200 pounds, which meant I had a lot more meat for my arms and legs to carry.

In the first twenty feet of my swim, someone kicked my head, my goggles flew off and I started to drown. I was saved by the lifeguard, who threw me a flotation device. Andrea, an accomplished swimmer, was already distancing herself from the pack. She had no idea what had happened to me. Meanwhile, I sat alone on the golden sand of Lake Lanier, my knees bent with my head lowered to my hands. As I sat there soaking in my new black bathing suit, sulking seemed the only logical response.

The year 2009 had been difficult, I thought. I'd had a lot of things to deal with. And now, the race I'd been training so hard for the last six months was slipping away.

That's when I told myself, "I have to do this."

I had wanted to complete the swim in fifteen minutes and do the event in record time, but I wasn't in shape to achieve those goals. Still, I wasn't going to let a rocky start prevent me from finishing the triathlon. In the past, I would have done this for other people with CF, but this was for me, and I wanted it badly. I remembered someone once telling me how easy it is to accomplish something great when life is wonderful, but how difficult it is to persevere when facing adversity. This was a true test to see if I could put my depression behind me. I put my goggles back on and re-entered the water.

Andrea cleaned my clock, completing the race in less than two hours. It was another amazing achievement for someone who battles multiple sclerosis. I did the swim in about forty-five minutes, completed the bike ride in an hour and finished the run in forty-five minutes. I huffed and puffed most of the way, and worried that my health was not up to par. I wanted to have a better time and was distraught from almost drowning, but days later I realized what a tremendous accomplishment completing a triathlon was—especially for someone with cystic fibrosis.

I ran the Peachtree Road Race a month later in eighty minutes. I was embarrassed that I had to walk instead of run up the hills. It was the first time in thirteen years that I'd walked any part of the Peachtree. My coughing had gotten much worse. The real kicker was that one of my friends thought that I had swapped my racing number with someone who was much older and out of shape. The reason he wondered this was that for the first time in Peachtree history our times were posted on the Internet and eighty minutes was not a time I normally registered. I was ashamed, and more importantly, worried about my health.

A few weeks later I got worse news. Dr. Wolfenden was diagnosed with breast cancer and would be out indefinitely. I'd have to see someone else. My numbers were down several percentage points and my new doctor, Dr. Viranuj Sueblinvong, told me that a stint on oral antibiotics was necessary. If my numbers didn't improve over the next three weeks, IV antibiotics would be the next step. Fortunately, I managed to improve my pulmonary function percentage a few points so I was able to avoid IV antibiotics this time around. Yet despite feeling better and adding another impressive accomplishment to my athletic résumé, something more sinister was lurking.

Chapter 44
My Other CF Symptom

As much as cystic fibrosis has affected me physically, it's had an even greater effect on my emotional state. Depression has always hovered above me, waiting to drop and crush me with little notice. Even worse, denial has been its constant companion.

For me, and thousands of others, depression and denial are symptoms of this horrible disease every bit as much as the breathing difficulty. The frightening thing about depression is that it never goes away. It hides, waiting for an incident to spark its return. The girl who walked in on me while I was doing my therapy is a perfect example. I thought I was doing fine. Things were getting better. Then she walked in and my life did a 180-degree turn.

Depression is an illness, a psychotic disorder marked by sadness, inactivity and self-depreciation, and usually accompanied by a reduction in activity and vitality. That dictionary definition, however, doesn't capture the intensity of the sadness and the roller-coaster of desperation and anxiety that are followed by periods of not caring about anything, or wishing it (life) would just go away.

Because I'd done things in my life that inspired others, I felt people saw me as a larger-than-life role model. I felt that image required me to be a super hero, constantly persevering and always positive, yet deep inside I knew that image was disingenuous. Because of the self-induced pressure to fit into this role, I never confronted my depression.

While having a life-threatening disease entitled me to some down moments, the unhealthy feelings I garnered over time became even more threatening. Without being fully aware of it, I let them conquer my emotions and my way of life. When good things happened to me, I used them to cover up my depression-hiding those dreadful feelings even from me. I didn't realize how full of self-hate I was. I thought the fact that I disliked talking about myself meant I was modest. Finally, I realized that it had nothing to do with being humble. I was battling severe clinical depression.

Intellectually, I knew that depression often affects people with chronic and life threatening illnesses, and deep down I knew I was in trouble. Practically, however, I just didn't know what to do about it.

Overwhelmed and unable to cope, I grew apart from my kids and my wife and did things to drive them away. Whenever Andrea needed something, I was unable to deliver. It was as if I were at the bottom of a well and could not escape. Each time I failed to come through for my family, the well grew deeper. I hurt Andrea with things I did and things I didn't do. What hurt her most was that I became a basement hermit, getting my happiness from social networking on the computer rather than my family. I spent my time "chatting" with other people instead of the woman and children I loved, using the Internet to escape thinking about my failures as a husband and father, and my concerns about our family's overall health.

The only way I knew to validate my worthiness was by acquiring as many friends as I could on Facebook and then bragging to others how many friends I had. It was as if I won the lottery when I surpassed a thousand friends. The truth was that I barely knew most of these people, and their positive comments gave me only temporary satisfaction. Moments later, I would fall right back into my dark existence. Andrea noticed the changes in me. I no longer laughed the way I once did. Nor did I respond with emotion during sad movies. I stopped telling my corny jokes. Andrea told me that she missed that side of me. I was, emotionally, dead. I could tell by Andrea's many questions about my emotional state that my stoic disposition frustrated and frightened her.

I told myself that my reactions were justified and normal. I had a sick son, I'd dealt with disease myself and things just continued to crumble in my life. I needed an escape and social networking with those who seemed to be in a similar predicament seemed to fill that role. I communicated with cystic fibrosis patients more than with my own parents. More than with my own kids. More than with my own wife.

I still spent entire days chatting on Facebook. I became addicted. I began living a virtual existence and was essentially living a double life. People saw me as an inspiring public speaker who worked hard for charity. In reality, I was a depressed Facebook junkie who could not get enough.

I'd been a "chatting" junkie even before the days of Facebook. Since I graduated from college, I coped with my depression by e-mailing others, seeking their positive comments. I thought I was coping better than my dark days in college. The truth was that I was just substituting one bad coping method for another.

Andrea, who in the past begged me to go to therapy, was more adamant this time. Our relationship became strained. She had nursed me when I was sick, sent me away on a great baseball trip, and helped give me two beautiful children. In exchange, I only did things that hurt her. Instead of appreciating the things she did for me, I looked at her sacrifices as more pressure on me. That's not to say that Andrea was perfect, but that's how depression warps a person's thoughts. My mindset was that everything I did was wrong and everything she did was right. I was a mess. I didn't know how to cope.

Faced with inner-conflict and guilt, I closed my Facebook account. While my next move should have been to fix things with my family, my concentration was somewhere else entirely. My focus turned towards ending my life.

I began reading about suicide on the Internet. I Googled a suicide prevention page that told me to think long and hard before making this fatal and final decision. The conflict inside me was terrible. I'd emotionally abandoned my family and didn't see the point of living another day. I'd been a hypocrite in many ways. At the same time, I couldn't purposely leave my children without a father and my wife without a husband, even knowing that for several months, I'd essentially done that. The night after my daughter's third birthday I cried in my mom's arms as she came over to console me. I had really hurt everyone in my family, especially Andrea, the woman I so deeply loved. I contemplated suicide and told my mom of my feelings.

"Stop it! You are not a terrible person. You've made mistakes. You can make things better. You have to fix yourself first."

It was as if my mom and I were having the conversation we should have had nearly thirty years ago, after I read the encyclopedia article that predicted I'd be dead by the age of twenty-five. My mom was the one person I could talk to because, emotionally, we're very much alike. I knew she felt guilt for not noticing my issues sooner, not being more open about things when I was younger, and being too over-protective of me when I needed to face the consequences of life. I don't blame my parents for my poor coping skills because I know they only wanted to protect me. I guess they assumed that one day I would protect myself, but I never learned to handle emotional things in a healthy way.

The next day, I went to a therapist who was able to help me deal with my issues. Tracy McConaghie and another therapist, George Rinker, whom I worked with later, said my poor coping skills could be attributed to the awful incidents that happened during the formative years of my youth.

In the past I'd been somewhat skeptical about "childhood incident psychology," but the more I talked with the therapist, the more I realized that many suppressed memories from the awkward sexual incidents with the family friend to being teased by classmates because I was weak and skinny, drove me to seek validation from Facebook friends even as I was ignoring my family. I kept telling myself that I was entitled to the praise I was getting from strangers. Truth be told, I had become addicted to digital praise. Like an alcoholic needs that one last drink, I needed one more kind word from someone I only knew through typing on a keyboard. This troubling compulsion became my fix. This addiction became the only way I could satisfy my feeling of unworthiness.

Keeping things quiet was how my family dealt with big issues and I used the same routine. The fact that I didn't know how to cope resulted in my refusal to take charge of any family needs. The unenviable task of taking on these responsibilities fell to Andrea. Reluctantly, she did all of our finances. She handled the insurance. She decided the kids' activities. She cleaned. She fixed up the house. I didn't do anything. My actions, or lack of actions, only infuriated Andrea more and caused hardship to our marriage.

While I was stuck in a world of depression and high anxiety, I was forced to mask my feelings. Ironically, I was still making motivational speeches to high schools and civic organizations and getting standing ovations and letters of gratitude from people I'd touched through my speeches and writings. I seemed to have no problem motivating others; the one person I could not seem to motivate was me. I didn't know what to do. I felt abandoned and unloved, and that I deserved this misery because I'd let down Andrea and so many friends and people who had looked up to me. It seemed I was flailing away with every attempt to regain the happiness I'd lost. I just wanted to end it all and disappear, but I knew I owed Andrea more than that. I thought I was making positive strides in therapy and I took a bigger part in day-to-day family errands. I took care of the children so Andrea could play tennis and go out with her friends, things she desperately needed and deserved. It also allowed me valuable one-on-one time with Avery and Ethan. They even sat with me while I did my therapy in the mornings. The one moment that touched me the most was one Saturday morning when the door opened and Avery announced, "Daddy, I missed you. I'll sit with you." She put her arms around me and gave me a hug. It was then that I knew that if I did not get better, I would lose those kinds of moments. I nearly cried as I gave Avery the biggest hug a guy in a pulsating vest could give. Sharing those moments with my children helped me forget the emotional highs of social networking.

Emily did her best to take things off my plate so I could focus on getting better. My sister became my co-chair at A Wish for Wendy and was amazing at creating fundraising events. Emily's ideas for Comedy for a Cure and Cocktails for a Cure helped raise more than five thousand dollars for A Wish for Wendy and the Cystic Fibrosis Foundation. She'd come a long way from being a reckless teenager.

Andrea and I went on dates and were becoming closer. Romance was starting to blossom again and her anger returned to love. I took Avery on father-daughter outings most weekends, which included trips to play miniature golf and riding the carousel at the mall. I wanted to make my family the priority they deserved to be. The transition wasn't easy. Initially, it felt unnatural to do errands around the house and spend so much time with my family, but the thanks I got in the form of hugs and kisses from my loved ones made the changes easier to accept.

I had what appeared to be good days, but in the end I wasn't healing like I should. Things seemed better on the outside, but inside I was still often anxious and depressed. I relapsed into conversing on-line again and ignoring the people I loved. I knew it was wrong and I knew it could cost me everything. That's the thing about addictions or compulsions. The consequences are obvious, but they won't stop you from risking everything good in your life. Andrea grew angry with me again. She said she had all but forgiven me but now we had to start over again. I didn't want to lose her, nor did I want to lose my two beautiful children. As a last resort, I checked into Ridgeview Institute, a mental hospital that dealt with depression and addiction. Fittingly, I arrived on Friday the thirteenth to be assessed. My life had become a horror movie in so many ways. I was admitted to the outpatient program three hours a day, five days a week for four weeks. My father took care of things in the office and allowed me to take a leave of absence.

My treatment began the following Tuesday. The first morning at Ridgeview, I filled out a ream of paperwork so I could admit myself. I'd realized when my father and I arrived at Ridgeview the prior Friday that the institute was on the same exit as the cemetery where my friend Jon and my sister Wendy were buried. It made me think of the dreams I'd had where my sister asked if I needed help. Here I was finally getting the help I needed and she was only a couple of miles away. I visited her and Jon three times in the four weeks that I was there.

Around 9:05 A.M. on November 17th, I arrived at the waiting area, moments before my first lecture. During our daily lectures we got into groups and participated in presentations that concerned self-esteem, conflict resolution and how to self-soothe. Afterward, we got a thirty-minute break during which most days I decided to go running. After the break I joined a group led by my caseworker, Jamie Singleteary, a young woman with great insight when it came to giving feedback. Our group was considered primary psych and secondary addiction, meaning that the focus was on our depression and anxiety, but we were able to deal with compulsive behaviors as well.

Every day started with fifteen minutes of meditation. Then came an hour lecture, and after the thirty-minute break, I attended group for an hour and a quarter. Problems among patients in my group ranged from drug abuse to severe anxiety. There was not a subject that was too taboo for this group. No one judged anyone else. No matter how strange a story seemed, we listened, gave feedback, and shared commonalities with our own illnesses. I found it horrifying that most issues these individuals dealt with were results of troubling events during their childhood. Patients admitted disturbing truths about their younger years that resulted in tearful episodes from every member of our group. It made me further examine my childhood traumas, but also realize how important it was to be a good role model for Ethan and Avery. We had to do three assignments before graduating. First was a self-assessment of our issues. The next was a timeline of everything that had happened in our life, including things that might have contributed to our problems. Finally, we had to produce a recovery plan that included what we'd learned from our stay and how we were going to approach our future without our "drug" of choice. My issues were depression and anxiety, complicated by addictive behaviors and compulsions. The compulsion to chat with people on-line had little to do with wanting to avoid my family, but, was rather, a result of being shamed most of my life. I simply wanted validation that I was worthy. I was a motivational speaker and scored eight out of thirty on the self-esteem test at Ridgeview. That's how bad my depression was. I scored one of the lowest, if not the lowest, in a forty-person class full of depressives, addicts, and people who were dealing with high anxiety. We were taught that everyone has similar thoughts. It's the kind of feelings that develop from those thoughts that distinguish a healthy person from a depressed person.

I met with Dr. Branko Radulovacki, or Dr. Rad as he was known at Ridgeview, the second day. He was a tall man with short hair and a slender build. He had a poker player's temperament, and never gave away what my answers meant to him. Dr. Rad added a new medication to my already long list, a drug to help with my depression. While at Ridgeview, I worked as hard as I'd ever worked for anything. I asked questions. I spoke up. I felt like I was back at school, only the subject I was studying wasn't math or science. I was learning about the inner-workings of Andy Lipman. We also had to attend twelve-step meetings while we were there. I attended a multi-family session with Andrea, where friends or family of the patient were included in the group and voiced their concerns. Andrea was the first one to speak. She cried about our issues, which was a step for her to heal.

A week later, I attended my first addiction meeting. Discussing my issues with the group and receiving their feedback helped me greatly. I've attended weekly meetings for more than a year.

Dr. Rad and I continued to work together; I saw him every other morning. He asked if I acted on desires or had temptations. I did not have temptations to e-mail on social networking sites, but I did miss the highs that I received from them. I missed feeling worthy, but I realized that only I could make myself be worthy. No e-mail in the world could serve that purpose. On my last day at Ridgeview, I was given a card from Jamie and the rest of my group wishing me well. I also received a serenity coin that I keep with me in case I feel the need for a high, or if I just need some comfort when I am depressed. The serenity prayer, printed on the coin, has become such a big part of my life that I have memorized it and repeat it morning and night as part of my prayer ritual.

I continue to see my therapist, George Rinker. Tracy did a wonderful job but I wanted someone who specializes in my issues. George is bringing a lot of my troubles back to the encounters with the daughter of my parents' friends. He tells me that's why I feel shame and seek worthiness. He's had a lot of patients like me and believes I can be cured. Until then, I will stay away from my triggers as much as possible. After several months of looking, I did eventually find the daughter of my parents' family friend. I also found the babysitter who beat me around that same time. I did some research on the girl and saw that she had her own mental issues and I felt confronting her was not worth pursuing. As far as the guy goes, I actually sent him an e-mail explaining why his actions so significantly hurt me. I never got a response. That's okay, I have finally closed the book on both of these childhood tragedies and now can focus on moving forward.

My biggest depression triggers include confrontation, boredom and winter. Winter may seem strange, but that always seems to be the time I get sick. It's also hard to exercise because night falls so fast and it's too cold to go out.

As far as the confrontation part goes, Andrea and I used to have arguments where I just cowered and let her be right. I remember both men and women telling me that once we got married the important thing was to say, "Yes, Dear." Truth be told, that was not good for me, nor was it beneficial to Andrea. I grew bitter and full of resentment. Andrea felt I wasn't interested or that I didn't think the issue was important enough to discuss. From my time at Ridgeview, I learned that I no longer could just agree to appease the woman I loved. I had to stand up for myself. That change of attitude not only helped me, it helped Andrea and our relationship.

I see Dr. Rad quarterly, along with attending support sessions once a month. The meetings bring together people who have let compulsive behavior and depression destroy their lives. We have a lot in common and learn a lot from each other. I've made some very healthy changes in my life. This time I'm confronting my issues rather than avoiding them. That's why I know that this time I will get better. I'm determined to keep a positive attitude, yet there always seems to be another challenge.

My next challenge materialized on a rainy Tuesday morning in February in the form of an e-mail from my nurse. She informed me that the results of a sputum culture test detected pseudomonas. Doctors had always been amazed I'd avoided this infection for so long, as most CF patients had it before their teens. I couldn't explain why I hadn't contracted it until now; perhaps it was because I was careful about things I touched and made sure people I hung out with weren't sick. I can't imagine that other patients were not just as careful. Perhaps I was fortunate. There are a myriad of ways to get pseudomonas and not knowing where I got it means there is a chance I can be exposed the same way again.

I always thought I'd be devastated to learn I had this infection, believing it would precede a quick sequence of being in a hospital, a transplant, and finally a coffin. Even when I got home that day, Andrea gave me a big hug and told me she was there for me. That was tough to hear in some ways, because I wanted her to focus on herself and what she needed to get better. I did not want my health scare to stall that process. At the same time, I realized that if I could show toughness this time around and not rely on the compliments of others, perhaps I could prove to her that I was a changed man.

I refused to pity myself this time and start the same old cycle again. This time things were going to be different. Over the past few months, I'd had time to analyze my life. I knew that to beat pseudomonas, I'd have to find that competitive spirit, my "Eye of the Tiger," and I did. I faithfully took the new medications my doctors prescribed, hired a personal trainer, and got into an even more rigorous workout routine. Instead of running a few miles a week, I ran five or six. Instead of doing two hours of treatments per day, I was doing close to four hours. In fact, I spent more time working out and doing treatments on an average day than I spent sleeping at night. Compared to beating depression, though, overcoming pseudomonas seemed easy. I had sputum samples tested regularly until they verified the pseudomonas was gone. Too bad there is no such test to assure patients that depression or addiction no longer lurks within.

Eventually, the culture results revealed that the antibiotics had killed the pseudomonas bug. Still, my pulmonary function scores were down, so I had to stay on the antibiotics and the three to four hours of treatments per day. I suppose it's better than the alternative of getting sicker and having even less valuable time with my children. After finding out that my cholesterol was in the "dangerous" range, I decided to embark on a new calorie-counting diet. I also stopped drinking sodas. In six months, I went from 203 pounds down to 180 pounds. My cholesterol improved seventeen percent in that time. As far as my emotional journey goes, I have been sober of my compulsive issues for nearly eighteen months. I have a sponsor for the meetings I attend and even have a sponsee, who I support.

I continue to worry about Andrea and feel guilt for causing her pain. We still have our difficult conversations, but conversation is the operative word. We are communicating for the first time in a long time. Slowly, she is building faith and trust in me again and slowly I'm learning how to live a worthy life while conquering my demons. My mom and I talk about my therapy sessions from time to time. She's interested and wants to help. It's difficult to talk about my innermost problems with my mom, so I simply discuss my feelings and what I learn from my sessions. I see my dad trying sometimes, but I don't know that he can empathize as much. My father is kind of like a general in the army. He doesn't put up with weakness or excuses. I only remember seeing him cry once. That was the day his mother passed away. So it's hard to break down around him, even though I know he loves me and I know he's taking steps to understand. He and my mom have attended meetings with me and the bond between us has gotten stronger.

I'm trying to use my mistakes as an opportunity not just to be a good father, but to be an incredible father. One day my kids will read about how their father ignored his family and hurt their mother for months on end. I want them to know that the mistakes I made never affected my love for them. I tell Avery and Ethan every night that I love them and can't wait to see them in the morning. I jump at the chance to put them to bed and kiss them every day when I leave for work. Andrea found a speech therapist for Ethan, as he is speech-delayed due to the stroke he suffered at birth. We had twenty percent of Ethan's cord blood—which we saved immediately after his birth—reinfused to hopefully heal the part of the brain affected by the stroke. This was done when Ethan was seven months old and while the results have been inconclusive overall, we believe the transfusion to be a tremendous success for our son. At three years old, he continues to improve and the smallest new gesture he makes or word he says is the highlight of most days for our family. Despite a negative prognosis at birth, Ethan has proven so many medical professionals wrong. I suppose that runs in the family. Avery, at five, sometimes talks to me as if she's the parent and I am the child. I tell her that I knew she would be a girl before she was born. While she may think I just happened to guess right, one day I will tell her about the aunt that she never met and hopefully she will realize my inkling was much more than a guess. Avery's only issue has been peanut allergies, which has required four trips to the emergency room. Parenting can be scary, but the rewards are great and the hard work is paying off. Avery and I have never been closer and Ethan is definitely a daddy's boy. Avery's fear of my therapy machine no longer exists, as every morning she and her brother come down to the basement to sit with me and watch television while I do my treatments. I'm lucky to have them and I hope they'll always feel the same way about their father.

As far as my friends go, Ross continues to be the best friend a guy could have. We try to meet for lunch at least once a week, as he works nearby. William Shields, my roommate at Georgia prior to living with Haim, has also become a great friend. We play tennis and get together for daddy-daughter breakfasts every now and then.

I did meet a new friend, Rusty Sneiderman. Rusty and his wife, Andrea, have become our closest couple friends. Rusty and I grab lunch weekly since we work about a mile from each other. We also hit the batting cage, the pool and occasional fundraising events. He and his wife invite us to their lake house often and, in exchange, we take them to Braves games. Rusty is the kind of guy anyone would feel lucky to be friends with. He is hard working, supportive and good-natured. His self-deprecating humor keeps me in hysterics.

My behavior affected a lot of people negatively. As I have gone through the process of psychological healing, I've had to re-examine my own life, and my expectations and my perception of myself. It always bothered me when people said, "I don't want to tell you my problems because you're an amazing person and you've dealt with far worse." While some might take a comment like that as a compliment, I took it as a reason I could never show imperfection or open up about the reasons for my depression. It meant I'd have to live in disguise forever. I thought I'd be disappointing those who looked to me for inspiration if I showed even an ounce of vulnerability.

I've learned to forgive myself for making mistakes, big or small, and to accept the fact that I'll never be anything close to perfect. The disguise is no longer necessary.

Another good thing about facing my depression and compulsion, besides the positive result it's had on my communication with Andrea and the additional time I spend with my family, is that I've realized that I'm not alone. I've had several people with CF tell me that they've been through these things and contemplated dark thoughts, too. The problem is so widespread that Dr. Wolfenden's office began doing surveys with young CF adults to catch depression and anxiety before it gets worse. Apparently, depression is a more common symptom of CF than previously thought. I wish I could talk to Dr. Wolfenden about this aspect of CF and how it has affected me, but that is no longer possible. Lindy Wolfenden, my doctor and friend, died of breast cancer in July of 2010, at the age of only forty. I was sad and heartbroken. Had she died prior to my treatment at Ridgeview, I'm sure I would have plunged into an even deeper depression. But I recognize now that death is part of life, and that over time the grieving will end, even though I will always miss her. Instead of growing more depressed from her loss, I used the memory of her spirit to show the world what an amazing doctor she was to me. The Wish for Wendy Challenge information table now bears her name, and her husband and two sons threw out the first pitch at the 11th annual tournament.

Meeting my peers at Ridgeview has greatly helped me as well. There are a lot of good people in this world who have allowed their depression and compulsions to cause them to behave inappropriately. There is still hope for all of them. I have to believe that, because I am one of them.

People still tell me from time-to-time that my bravery and hard work inspire them. Now, though, instead of living in a disguise of perfection, I'm more open. It reminds me when Rusty and I were having a conversation and he told me he was embarrassed to tell me his problems because I'd dealt with far worse. My response was simple.

"Hey, believe me when I say I'm like everyone else. I make mistakes and I pay for them. Perspective is different for everyone. We all have our issues. We just have to work hard to correct them."

I have learned to deal with my emotional shortcomings and how to turn them into strengths. That's not to say that I have not struggled with this adjustment. I'm not immune to the negative effects that depression can bring to my life, but I am more aware of them now and I have mental weapons to combat them. I realize that like CF, these issues can serve as a platform to make others aware of the warning signs of clinical depression. I now not only share my accomplishments during my speeches, but I also talk about my fight against depression. While days go by and I celebrate Facebook sobriety milestones, I realize that like depression and probably cystic fibrosis, addiction will be a battle I will have to fight my entire life. That is why I take just as much pride in beating these two emotional ailments as I do conquering cystic fibrosis. After all, facing and beating my emotional nemesis might be my biggest accomplishment yet. It may be even greater than beating the terminal lung disease that has tormented me my entire life.

Chapter 45
Wishing I Was More Rusty

As a speaker, the one comment I never wanted to hear was, "You seemed a bit rusty." I heard it a few times presenting for my Toastmasters group when I first began public speaking. They made fun of my grammar and I was fine. They commented on how many times I said "um..." and I could deal with that. They even said they didn't understand the point of my speech and I could handle that, but if I heard, "You seemed a bit rusty," I got really frustrated. To me it meant that I wasn't working at my craft and I knew I worked hard when it came to my passion for public speaking.

During the time I suffered most acutely from clinical depression, my passion for motivational speaking diminished. Through the years, two people really pushed me to make my speaking more of a priority. One was my father. The other was my friend, Rusty.

While Rusty and I had only known each other for two years, we had become great friends. Andrea and I met Rusty, his Andrea, and their kids Sophia and Ian, at a friend's party. Soon afterward, we were as inseparable as the Flintstones and Rubbles. As our couple friendship developed, the Andreas (Rusty and I had to use the terms "My Andrea" or "Your Andrea" to avoid confusion) became even closer, as did Rusty and I.

Rusty and I talked pretty regularly. He once told me that it was nice to be friends with a couple both he and his wife liked individually. During our many lunches in Duluth, where we both worked, Rusty concluded every encounter with a question, "Now how can I help you to be more of a success." I remember the first time he came to dinner and he said he wanted to repay us for making the meal. So what did he do? He went outside and fixed our gutter. The man got his masters at Harvard, was a brilliant businessman and the CFO of a big company, and here he was fixing our gutter. That's when I knew I found a one-in-a-million type friend.

Rusty was a big fan of mine for some reason. He told me that I inspired him and he told my parents that he loved me and would do whatever I wanted to help make Wish for Wendy a success. He believed in me and, in turn, I believed in him. Rusty was always hungry for success. He wanted to make a difference.

Rusty played on the only two foundation teams we've ever had and agreed to take on the heavy responsibility of being our sponsorship chairman in 2010 and for many years to come. He came up with some great ideas and helped us find several new corporate sponsors.

Rusty had an amazing personality and sense of humor. He was known for making fun of his athletic activity, though he was no slouch, as he proved on the softball field. He once bought a Wii FIT and said after he took the fitness test that the Wii told him that his fitness was equal to that of a grossly obese seventy-five-year-old. Rusty laughed, "I paid money for a machine to tell me I'm old and fat. No thank you!"

The 2010 Wish for Wendy Warriors foundation team had a lot of new names, but one name stayed the same—Rusty Sneiderman. Rusty played softball once a year and this was it. Rusty was always introducing me to people he thought could help my career and/or my foundation. He got along with every person I introduced him to. My parents really loved him. He and my dad had the same bug about starting a business on their own. They talked frequently.

Though Rusty and I had only known each other for two years, we talked about growing old and all of the trips we were going to take together. We each had two children, a girl first and then a boy. The kids were almost the same age. We talked about his next business venture and how he was really excited to get started. No matter how much a lunch was full of talking about his business, it always ended with, "Now, how I can I help you to be successful."

Rusty was my biggest blog fan. I created a blog in 2009 and Rusty was its most avid reader. He would literally read every passage I wrote and talk to me about it every time he saw me. He encouraged me to better myself. He told me that my story could help people who were suffering from depression. He wanted to create a plan to help me. The man was starting up a business, was married, was raising two children and had many charitable obligations, yet he always wanted to help me. I wish I'd taken him up on it...at least in the professional sense.

On a Thursday in mid-November 2010, I was working on my book—coincidentally, another project Rusty encouraged me to finish in order to help others—when my wife called. She was crying. My first thought was something happened to one of the kids.

"Rusty's been shot," she said. "WHATTTTTT?" I said. "Where, when, how..." Rusty was one of the least violent people I knew; surely this was a mistake. Half an hour earlier Russell J. Sneiderman had walked out of a preschool in a very safe part of north Atlanta after dropping off his son and was shot several times at close range. An hour later, he was declared dead.

My mom, dad, Andrea and I were at the hospital. Andrea was a real rock for Rusty's Andrea. Many of Andrea Sneiderman's friends came to support her. The story became national news. With Rusty's family's permission, I did some interviews with a couple of the local stations in order to paint a picture of my good friend. The prevailing question from everyone who was fortunate to have Rusty Sneiderman as a friend was, "Why? Why would someone do this to such an amazing man?" I can tell you that the police found the man who did this and that Rusty did nothing to deserve what happened to him.

Rather than talk about Rusty's death, I'd prefer to remember his life and our friendship. It was an honor to know Rusty Sneiderman. He wasn't just a friend. He was a best friend. He wasn't just a guy who gave to charity; he contributed to causes to help them to become successful. I'm richer for having known Rusty.

Rusty always told me that I inspired him. I wish I'd had time to tell him what an amazing friend he was to me. I loved Rusty like a brother. I miss him so much. I will do all I can to honor his memory because he believed in me.

On a dismal Sunday morning in November, I gave the biggest speech of my life. Rusty would have wanted me to do that. The speech was Rusty's eulogy. I had to say goodbye to a man that should still be here. I had to say goodbye to a man who will miss out on so many amazing things because of one pure evil act. I had to say goodbye to a man whom I planned to spend so much time with over the next few decades. I thought how ironic it was that Rusty pointed out to me that I had reached the 2010 median life expectancy of someone with CF when I turned 37. He was very proud of me. When I was born, there were not a lot of people who would have guessed I would have reached 37. The sad thing is that Rusty died at 36 and, sadly, it was he who would never see his 37th birthday.

We lost an amazing man, father, son, brother, husband and a friend. Rusty always had dreams of being a big success and making a difference. Little did he know that he accomplished both missions. He made everyone around him better. That's the greatest success one man can have. I will honor him, as will so many others, till the day we die.

I continue to battle depression and losing Rusty sure didn't help. However, I use the tools I learned at Ridgeview and depend on my sponsor and therapist to get through the tough days. I have even met with my rabbi. I still have flashbacks of my adventures with Rusty. I remember the first time we went to a Braves game. I remember his words of encouragement when we shared a lunch together. I remember his infectious smile and the way he made me feel. Those memories will never fade.

I plan to honor Rusty by being the best speaker I can be and relaying my message to other people who could truly benefit from it. And the next time I hear that comment that once infuriated me, my reaction will be a little different. I can just hear it now.

"Andy, you seemed a bit Rusty."

God, I hope so...I really hope so.

Epilogue

The cystic fibrosis gene was discovered nearly two decades ago, but there is still no cure. Until recently, there have not been any drugs to correct the genetic defect in CF patients. In 2011, Vertex Pharmaceuticals announced that the drug VX-770 improved lung function in people with cystic fibrosis, some by as much as ten percent. The drug also reduced the frequency of disease exacerbations that required treatment with antibiotics.

Doctors stop short of saying this drug will cure cystic fibrosis, but it certainly qualifies as a breakthrough. I stopped believing there would ever be a cure several years ago. I stopped picturing myself without cystic fibrosis. I stopped envisioning a "normal" life. It is the only way that I can avoid disappointment. I hope one day that researchers can make me believe again.

In fact, there are positive developments. For example, the current median life expectancy for CF patients of 37 years is an all-time high. I recently turned 38, which was particularly important for me since that meant for the first time in my life I was ahead of the life expectancy statistics.

There were no role models with cystic fibrosis when I was growing up, and there were so few adults with cystic fibrosis that they didn't even have adult centers. Men over the age of twenty at a CF clinic were assumed to be the father of a child with cystic fibrosis, not a patient. Breakthrough treatments were only rumors. In the CF world, hope was nonexistent.

As I grew older, I thought back to the days of my early twenties and prayed no one would ever feel as hopeless as I did then. I hoped it wouldn't take someone else with CF the twenty years it took me to figure out that life was worth living. No one should ever have to live in fear of cystic fibrosis, or any other disability or disease. Life deals each of us a different hand but, like poker, it's not always the hand you're dealt that matters, it's what you do with that hand. I have tried to take advantage of my position as a thriving patient with cystic fibrosis. In 2011, I became the first cystic fibrosis patient to serve on the board of the Georgia Chapter of the Cystic Fibrosis Foundation. As I promised Rusty, I increased the number of speeches I made and spoke to the Cystic Fibrosis Pharmacy in Washington, D.C.

I fully recognized what was in the hand I'd been dealt at the A Wish for Wendy Softball Challenge in 2007. Andrea was talking to a man about our age who had been walking by with his son. He asked about the event because he had seen a sign saying it benefited the Cystic Fibrosis Foundation and told her his son had CF. Andrea introduced me to the man, and he introduced me to his four-year old son. The father looked at me and then back at him and said, "Toby, look at Mr. Lipman here. You can be strong, just like him."

Looking at the boy, my thoughts returned to the day I first saw the poster of a man in amazing physical condition. His self-confidence resonated from the poster. I remembered what my mother said: "He has cystic fibrosis. Look how strong he is."

Today, I realize the man in the poster could not have had cystic fibrosis. No one lived that long with CF back then and, even if they did, they didn't look like that. But, at eight years old, I didn't know any differently, so I believed. For many years, I continued to believe this man was real because I needed the inspiration. My mom gave me hope that day, hope that—as unrealistic as it seemed—there was a chance I could be that guy. I asked my mom about it recently and she had completely forgotten the incident. It's funny how sometimes the smallest things we do can have such enormous lasting effects on another person.

So when I saw the way Toby looked at me, I remembered being the little boy who wanted to believe in something. The difference was that Toby didn't have to look at a fictitious poster to know that he'd be all right. He could look at a living, breathing version of that model. I had become the man in the poster.

I hoped I could say something that would affect the little boy positively. "Toby," I said. "Be strong. Be a fighter. Then I gave Toby a book in which I scribbled a note with my favorite mantra: "Live your dreams and love your life."

I could see how much it meant to his father as he smiled at me and then at his son. I could already see the father's attitude change. He seemed proud, as if this moment signified the beginning of Toby's march towards greatness. I gave Toby one of the bright yellow softballs from our tournament and told his father that his son would be fine, because he had role models who have battled the same disease he battles. A lot of things had changed since I was a boy.

Maybe that's my role. Maybe I saw that poster for a reason. Maybe I was destined to help young children with cystic fibrosis realize their dreams. While cystic fibrosis wadded up most of my dreams and tossed them in the garbage when I was young, it has been a positive factor in the things I'm doing today. I don't know that I'd be raising money for any cause if I hadn't been affected by CF. I doubt I would have written a book or been nominated to run with the Olympic Torch. I probably would not be working so hard at staying healthy if it hadn't been for this disease.

In some weird way, cystic fibrosis has made my life better. It has given my life a purpose. It has helped me appreciate the little things more. Today, I'm okay with being a little different. And I'm okay with not having a normal life. I still have to battle the physical demands of the disease and be careful not to fall back into my depression, but I feel fortunate because I realize how lucky I am—how lucky we all are—to have a life at all.

Statistics can measure a lot of things, but I have learned that they can never measure a person's heart. No matter what your abilities or disabilities, rejoice in them, for there you can learn and grow. But, most importantly of all, there you can find all of your dreams.

About the Author

Andy Lipman has cystic fibrosis, but cystic fibrosis does not have him. Instead, Andy is a positive role model who defied all odds to become a college graduate, Olympic-torch bearer, 10K runner, husband, and father. He is dedicated to finding a cure for this genetic disease. Andy was born in Atlanta, Georgia, the second child of Charles and Eva Lipman, a businessman and former teacher turned stay-at-home-mom. Their first child, a beautiful daughter they named Wendy, also had cystic fibrosis but, unlike Andy, she lived only sixteen days.

Andy battled several traumatic episodes while a young boy that still affect him today. He spent many sickly childhood days trapped by uncomfortable breathing therapies, and was ridiculed and shunned by other children. Sports, along with Andy's determined spirit, changed all that. By the time he was in high school, he was considered an accomplished athlete. Whether he realized it or not, Andy's high level of physical fitness went a long way toward saving his life every time cystic fibrosis symptoms threatened.

While some people live to work out, in Andy's case, he works out in order to live. College, however, was another story. Overwhelmed by social pressures and class work, Andy became depressed, stopped taking his medication, and almost died. But his competitive nature kicked in and he took control of his life. When another CF related crisis came along his senior year, he battled it as hard as he'd fought anyone or anything. After college, a stint as a top salesman for Enterprise Rent-a-Car was followed by a day carrying the Olympic torch, numerous 10K runs, and meeting his wife, Andrea. He and Andrea managed to have two children, despite the fact that almost all men with cystic fibrosis are unable to have children, and the fact that Andrea is a cancer survivor who also has multiple sclerosis. Their failures and successes going through in vitro fertilization are well documented in his book. Several bouts of very serious illness and depression were headed off by Andy's unwavering zest for life and he founded the Wish For Wendy Foundation to both honor his older sister and to raise funds and awareness for cystic fibrosis and its cure.

Andy speaks regularly to students, civic and professional groups and associations about CF. His dynamic presentations are emotional and heartfelt, and he takes his position as a role model for children who have cystic fibrosis very seriously. He wants each of them to know that this disease does not have to be a death sentence and that they, too, can live lives fuller than anyone ever envisioned. Andy Lipman lives in Atlanta with his wife and two cherished children.